Lecture Notes in Artificial Intel

Subseries of Lecture Notes in Computer Sci
Edited by J. G. Carbonell and J. Siekmann

T0250638

Lecture Notes in Computer Science

Edited by G. Goos, J. Hartmanis, and J. van Leeuwen

Springer
Berlin
Heidelberg
New York
Hong Kong
London
Milan
Paris
Tokyo

Petra Perner (Ed.)

Advances
in Data Mining

Applications in E-Commerce, Medicine, and Knowledge Management

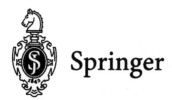

Springer

Series Editors

Jaime G. Carbonell, Carnegie Mellon University, Pittsburgh, PA, USA
Jörg Siekmann, University of Saarland, Saarbrücken, Germany

Volume Editor

Petra Perner
Institute of Computer Vision and Applied Science
August-Bebel-Str. 16-20
04275 Leipzig, Germany
E-mail: ibaiperner@aol.com

Cataloging-in-Publication Data applied for

Die Deutsche Bibliothek - CIP-Einheitsaufnahme

Advances in data mining : applications in E-commerce, medicine, and
knowledge management / Petra Perner (ed.). - Berlin ; Heidelberg ; New York ;
Barcelona ; Hong Kong ; London ; Milan ; Paris ; Tokyo : Springer, 2002
  (Lecture notes in computer science ; 2394 : Lecture notes in artificial
intelligence)
  ISBN 3-540-44116-6

CR Subject Classification (1998): I.2.6, I.2, H.2.8, K.4.4, J.3

ISSN 0302-9743
ISBN 3-540-44116-6 Springer-Verlag Berlin Heidelberg New York

Springer-Verlag Berlin Heidelberg New York
a member of BertelsmannSpringer Science+Business Media GmbH

http://www.springer.de

© Springer-Verlag Berlin Heidelberg 2002
Printed in Germany

Typesetting: Camera-ready by author, data conversion by PTP-Berlin Stefan Sossna e.K.
Printed on acid-free paper   06/3111   5 4 3 2 1

Preface

This book presents papers describing selected projects on the topic of data mining in fields like e-commerce, medicine, and knowledge management. The objective is to report on current results and at the same time to give a review on the present activities in this field in Germany. An effort has been made to include the latest scientific results, as well as lead the reader to the various fields of activity and the problems related to them.

Knowledge discovery on the basis of web data is a wide and fast-growing area. E-commerce is the principal theme of motivation in this field, as companies invest large sums in the electronic market, in order to maximize their profits and minimize their risks. Other applications are telelearning, teleteaching, service support, and citizen-information systems. Concerning these applications, there is a great need to understand and support the user by means of recommendation systems, adaptive information systems, as well as by personalization. In this respect Giudici and Blanc present in their paper procedures for the generation of associative models from the tracking behavior of the user. Perner and Fiss present in their paper a strategy for intelligent e-marketing with web mining and personalization. Methods and procedures for the generation of associative rules are presented in the paper by Hipp, Güntzer, and Nakhaeidizadeh.

The fast increase in information from the Human Genome Project on the one hand and new methods of genome-wide differential expression analysis, target-oriented manipulation of signal paths, and proteome research on the other hand has made it possible to study, far beyond a linear presentation of individual signal paths, the complex processing of signals in cells and their physiological as well patho-physiological importance. For the evaluation of the data generated, increasingly intelligent evaluation procedures are needed. Glass and Karopka describe in their paper methods for the evaluation of genomic expression data based on case-based reasoning. Another medical approach based on case-based reasoning for the prognosis of threatening influenza waves is described in the paper by Schmidt and Gierl.

Besides all cultural aspects, the field of knowledge management is especially concerned with the acquisition and extraction of knowledge from various sources and for different purposes. Data mining is an approach that very well supplements other knowledge management techniques. It enables automated knowledge extraction and evaluation from data bases, from intra-/internet, and from documents. Althoff et al. describe in their paper results of the indiGo project for expierence management and process learning and compare their results to related work on knowledge management.

All papers were presented at the second Industrial Conference on Data Mining ICDM 2002 in Leipzig. We would like to thank all those who contributed to this special event.

May 2002   Petra Perner

Table of Contents

Sequence Rules for Web Clickstream Analysis

Erika Blanc and Paolo Giudici

Department of Economics and Quantitative Methods
University of Pavia
Via San Felice 5, 27100 Pavia (Italy)
blaner@eco.unipv.it, giudici@unipv.it

Abstract. We present new methodologies for the search of sequence rules in the analysis of web clickstream data. We distinguish direct and indirect sequence rules, and show how to draw data mining conclusions on the basis of them. We then compare sequence rules, which are local models, with a global probabilistic expert system model. Our analysis have been conducted on a real e-commerce dataset.

1 Clickstream Analysis

Every time an user links up at a web site, the server keeps track of all the actions accomplished in the *log file*. What is captured is the "click flow" (click-stream) of the mouse and the keys used by the user during the navigation inside the site. Usually at every click of the mouse corresponds the visualization of a web page. Therefore, we can define a click-stream as the sequence of the requested pages.

The succession of the pages shown by a single user during his navigation inside the Web identifies an user session. Typically, the analysis only concentrates on the part of each user session concerning the access at a specific site. The set of the pages seen, inside a user session, coming from a determinate site is known with the term server session or, it is more commonly said that they identify a visit (J. Srivastava *et al.*, 2000).

We remark that other statistical methods can be applied to web clickstream data, in order to detect association rules. For instance, Blanc and Giudici (2002) consider, besides sequence rules, odds ratios and graphical loglinear models, while Blanc and Tarantola (2002) consider bayesian networks and dependency networks. Furthermore, in a recent paper, Di Scala and La Rocca (2002) also consider the application of Markov chain models to web data, with main emphasis on assessing homeogenity of the considered Markov chain. Finally, Rognoni, Giudici e Polpettini (2002) consider using Markov chains to estimate directly the transition probabilities from one page to another.

2 The Available Data

The data set that we consider for the analysis is the result of the elaboration of a log file concerning a site of e-commerce. The source of the data cannot be specified; however it is the website of a company that sells hardware and software products; it will be referred to as "a webshop". The accesses to the website have been registered in a logfile for a period of about two years, since 30 september 1997 to 30 june 1999. The logfile has then been processed to produce a dataset, named "sequences". Such dataset contains the user id (c_value), a variable with the date and the instant the visitor has linked to a specific page (c_time) and the web page seen (c_caller). Table 1 reports a small extract of the available dataset , corresponding to one visit.

Table 1. The considered dataset.

c_value	c_time	c_caller	c_order
70ee683a6df...	14OCT97:11:09:01	home	1
70ee683a6df...	14OCT97:11:09:08	catalog	2
70ee683a6df...	14OCT97:11:09:14	program	3
70ee683a6df...	14OCT97:11:09:23	product	4
70ee683a6df...	14OCT97:11:09:24	program	5

Table 1 describes that the visitor corresponding to the identifier (cookie) 70ee683a6df... has entered the site on the fourteenth of october, 1997, at 11:09:01, and has visited, in sequence, the pages home, catalog, program, product, program, leaving the website at 11:09:24.

The whole data set contains 250711 observations, each corresponding to a click, that describe the navigation paths of 22527 visitors among the 36 pages which compose the site of the webshop. The visitors are taken as unique, that is, no visitors appears with more than one session. On the other hand, we remark that a page can occurr more than once in the same session.

This data set is a noticeable example of a transactional dataset. It can be used directly, in a form as in Table 1, with as many rows as the number of total clicks, to determine association and sequence rules. Alternatively, a derived dataset can be used, named "visitors". It is organised by sessions, and contains variables that can characterise each of such sessions. These variables include important quantitative ones, such as the total time length of the server session (*length),* the total number of clicks made in a session (*clicks*), and the time in which the session starts (*start*, setting at 0 the midnight of the preceeding day). More importantly for our analysis, such dataset contains binary variables that describe whether each page is visited at least once (modality 1) or not (modality (0). Finally, there is a bianry variable, named purchase, that indicates whether the session has led to (at least) one e-commerce transaction.

Table 2 shows part of a row from the visitors dataset, that corresponds to the session in Table 1.

Table 2. The derived dataset.

c_value	c_time	length	clicks	time	home
70ee683a6df...	14OCT97:11:09:01	24	5	11:09:01	1

c_value	catalog	addcart	program	product
70ee683a6df...	1	0	1	1

While the rows in Table 1 correspond to clicks, in table 2 the rows correspond to sessions (or, equivalently, visitors, as they are unique). There are as many rows as the total number of visits to the web site. In particular, looking at the last five columns, it is obtained a binary data matrix that expresses which pages, among the 36 considered, have been visited at least once in each session.

To give an idea of the type of considered pages, we now list some among the most frequent ones.

HOME: the home page of the web site;

LOGIN: where a user has to enter its name and other personal information, during the first registration, in order to access to certain services and products, reserved to the customers;

LOGPOST: prompts a message that informs whether the login has been successful or if it has failed;

LOGOUT: on this page the user can leave the personal characterisation given in the login page;

REGISTER: in order to be later recognized, the visitor has to prompt a userid and password;

REGPOST: shows the partial results of the registration, asking for missing information;

RESULTS: once the registration is accomplished, this page summarizes the information given;

REGFORM1: here the visitor has to insert data that enable him/her to buy a product, such as a personal identification number;

REGFORM2: here the visitor has to subscribe a contract in which he/she accepts the conditions for on-line commerce HELP: it answers questions that may arise during the navigation through the web site;

FDBACK: a page that allows to go back to the previous one visited

FDPOST: a page that allows to go back to one previously seen page, in determined areas of the site

NEWS: it presents the last novelties available;

SHELF: it contains the list of the programs that can be downloaded from the website

PROGRAM: gives detailed information on the characteristics of the software programs that can be bought;

PROMO: gives an example (demo) of the peculiarities of a certain program;

DOWNLOAD: it allows to download software programs of interest;

CATALOG: it contains a complete list of the products on sale in the web site;

PRODUCT: shows detailed information on each product that can be purchased;

P_INFO: a page on which detailed information on the terms of payment of the products can be found;

ADDCART: the place where the virtual basket can be filled with items to be purchased;

CART: shows the current status of the basket, that is, which items it contains;

MDFYCART: allows to modify the current content of the basket, for instance taking off items;

CHARGE : indicates the amount due to buy the items contained in the basket;

PAY_REQ: a page which visualizes the amount finally due for the products in the basket;

PAY_RES: here the visitor agrees to pay, and data for payment are inserted (for example, the credit card number);

FREEZE: where the requested payment can be suspended, for instance to add new products to the basket.

3 Exploratory Data Analysis

Our main aim is to discover the most frequent sequence rules among the 36 binary variables describing whether any single page has been visited. In order to obtain valid conclusions, the considered data have to be homogeneous. In order to assess whether the visitors dataset (and, correspondingly, the sequence dataset that generates it) is homogeneous we have deemed necessary to run first an exploratory analysis on the visitors dataset. The available quantitative variables, which are somehow ancillary for the analysis, can be usefully employed for this purpose.

On the basis of the explanatory analysis, we have decided to proceed with outliers removal. We have decided to eliminate all observations above the 99-th percentile of the distribution of the variables *clicks* and *length*, which indeed behave similarly. On the other hand, we have decided not to remove observations possibly outlying with respect to the start variable. This because of the nature of the variable itself as well as the observed distribution.

The resulting visitors dataset contains 22152 observations, in place of the initial 22527.

In consideration of the heterogeneous nature of the navigators of the site, confirmed by the exploratory stage, we have decided to perform a cluster analysis, in order to find homogeneous clusters of behaviours. We remark that our primary goal here is not cluster analysis per se and, thus, cluster analysis can be seen as somehow exploratory or, better, preliminary, to the local models that we are seeking.

As clustering variables we have considered the three quantitative variables start, length, clicks, as well as the binary variable purchase, which can all be seen as instrumental to our objective, of understanding navigation patterns. For the cluster analysis, we have decided to first run a hierarchical method, to find the number of groups, and then a non-hierarchical method, to allocate observations in the determined number of groups. As distance function we have considered the Euclidean distance; as hierarchical method the method of Ward (after some comparative experiments). Finally, to allocate observations we have chosen the K-means non-hierarchical method.

Table 3 summarizes the results of the analysis, showing , for each cluster, its numerosity and the mean values of the four variables used in the classification. Notice that, for the purchase variable, the mean represents the proportion of actual purchases.

From Table 3 notice that there are two bigger groups, 1 and 4, with the other two smaller. We remark that, from this final cluster allocation, $R^2 = 59\%$, which indicates a good performance, given the complexity of the data at hand.

The results obtained from cluster analysis confirm heterogeneity of behaviours. To the purpose of finding navigation patterns, we have decided to concentrate the analysis on only one cluster. The choice has fallen on the third cluster. This choice is obviously subjective but, nevertheless, has two important peculiarities. First, the visitors in this cluster stay connected for long time, and visit many pages. Both these occurrences allow to better explore the navigation sequences between the web pages. Second, this cluster has a high probability of purchase; it seems important to consider the typical navigation pattern of a group of high purchasers.

Therefore, in the following sections, we shall consider a reduced dataset, corresponding to the third cluster, with 1240 sessions and 21889 clicks. Figure 1 gives, for such cluster, the percentages of visit to each single pages, and Figure 2 gives the corresponding pie diagram.

Before starting with the modelling results we remark that we have appended, in the cluster dataset, a start_session and an end_session page, respectively, before the first page and the last page visited in each session. Obviously, such pages are fictitious, and are not random, but certain. They will serve though to evidentiate the most common entrance and exit pages.

Table 3. Results from the cluster analysis.

Cluster	N. records	Variable	Cluster average	Total average
1	8802	Clicks	8	10
		Length	6 minutes	10 minutes
		Start	h. 18	h. 14
		Purchase	0.034	0.072
2	2859	Clicks	22	10
		Length	17 minutes	10 minutes
		Start	h. 15	h. 14
		Purchase	0.241	0.072
3	1240	Clicks	18	10
		Length	59 minutes	10 minutes
		Start	h. 13	h. 14
		Purchase	0.194	0.072
4	9251	Clicks	8	10
		Length	6 minutes	10 minutes
		Start	h. 10	h. 14
		Purchase	0.039	0.072

Field Details:

Field Name: C_CALLER

Category	Size %		Category	Size %
start_session	05,0937		modifycart	00,5915
home	07,9855		news	00,4354
program	10,7706		fdback	00,3040
product	17,9346		logout	00,2958
end_session	05,0937		download	02,6290
catalog	05,2539		regform	00,0041
p_info	07,0449		regform2	00,1438
register	02,5920		charge	00,0657
regpost	02,0703		fdpost	00,1232
shelf	03,2986		regform1	00,4026
addcart	03,8408		xfreeze	00,0863
cart	02,6454		promo	00,1191
freeze	04,6007		archive	00,0452
pay_req	03,6107		archdownload	00,0041
agb	00,5463		trial	00,0698
help	00,8133		freeze.new	00,0205
result	00,7353		payit	00,0534
login	04,6623		Missing	00,0000
logpost	03,5204		Invalid	00,0000
pay_res	02,4934			

Fig. 1. Description of the cluster data.

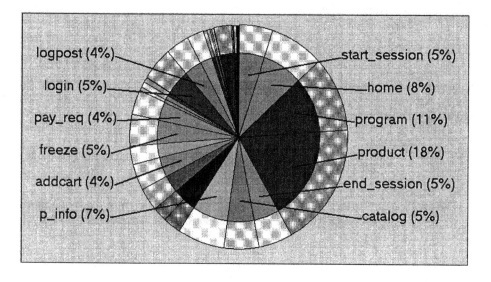

Fig. 2. Description of the cluster variables.

4 Indirected Sequence Rules

An association rule is a statement between two itemsets A and B, that can be written in the form A → B. If the rule is ordered in time we have a sequence rule: in this case

A preceeds B. For an introduction see, for example, Hastie, Tibshirani and Friedman (2001).

In web clickstream analysis, a sequence rule is typically indirect: namely, between the visit of page A and the visit of page B other pages can be seen. On the other hand, in a direct sequence rule A and B are seen consecutively.

In this paragraph we shall consider indirect rules; direct ones will be considered in the next paragraph.

A sequence rule model is, essentially, an algorithm that searches for the most interesting rules in a database.

The indexes commonly used in Web Mining to evaluate the importance of a sequence rule are the indexes of support and confidence.

Consider the indirect sequence $A \rightarrow B$ and indicate as $N_{A \rightarrow B}$ the number of visits which appear in such sequence, at least once. Let N be the total number of the server sessions. Notice that the rule $A \rightarrow B$ will be counted only once even if it had been repeated several times inside the session.

The support for the rule $A \rightarrow B$ is obtained dividing the number of server sessions which satisfy the rule by the total number of server sessions:

$$support\{A \rightarrow B\} = \frac{N_{A \rightarrow B}}{N} \tag{1}$$

Therefore, it is a relative frequency that indicates the percentage of the users that have visited in succession the two pages. In presence of a high number of visits, as it usually happens, it is possible to state that the support for the rule expresses the probability an user session contains the two pages in sequence:

$$support\{A \rightarrow B\} = \Pr\{A \rightarrow B\} \tag{2}$$

The confidence for the rule $A \rightarrow B$ instead is obtained dividing the number of server sessions which satisfy the rule by the number of sessions containing the page A:

$$confidence\{A \rightarrow B\} = \frac{N_{A \rightarrow B}}{N_A} = \frac{\frac{N_{A \rightarrow B}}{N}}{\frac{N_A}{N}} = \frac{support\{A \rightarrow B\}}{support\{A\}} \tag{3}$$

Therefore, the confidence approximates the conditional probability that in a server session in which has been seen the page A is subsequently required page B.

What just said has been referred to itemsets A and B containing one page each; however, each itemset can contain more than one page, and the previous definition stil hold. The order of a sequence is the total number of pages involved in the rule. The rules discussed so far are sequences of order two.

The main limit of the indexes of support and confidence, for other aspects extremely flexible and informative, is that, as descriptive indexes, they allow only to draw valid conclusions for the observed data set. In other terms, they do not allow to obtain some reliable behaviour forecasts for new users.

In particular, we have implemented our analysis in the software IBM Intelligent Miner for data, which is based on the calculation of the support as main interestingness measure of a sequence rule. The results obtained with Intelligent Miner for indirect sequences of two pages are shown in table 4; notice that the sequences have been ordered on basis of their support.

Table 4. The most frequent indirect sequences of order two.

Support (%)	Itemsets
100	start_session→end_session
88.790	start_session→product
88.790	product→end_session
77.661	start_session→program
77.661	program→end_session
73.387	program→product
64.677	product→product
62.097	start_session→home

From table 4 notice that the most supported rule is, obviously start_session → end_session, which is certain. We then have, among the most supported rules, those that indicate which are the most frequent referral (entrance) pages. These are the rules that start with the page start_session. The figure indicates that the most frequent entrance pages are product, program and home. Similarly, the rules with end_session as head of the rule indicate the most frequent exit pages. In the table we have that such pages are program and product.

Finally, the figure also indicates sequence rules between pages different from start_session and end_session: these are program → product and product → product.

Table 5 contains the most supported sequences of order greater than two. For the sake of clarity we have restricted them to those containing no more than 4 pages.

Table 5. The most frequent indirect sequences of order not higher than four.

Support (%)	Itemsets
100	start_session→end_session
88.790	product→end_session
88.790	start_session→product
88.790	start_session→product→end_session
77.661	program→end_session
77.661	start_session→program→end_session
77.661	start_session→program
73.387	program→product
73.387	start_session→program→product→end_session
73.387	start_session→program→product
73.387	program→product→end_session

From table 5 notice that many entering visitors see program or product.

5 Direct Sequence Rules

We now consider direct sequence rules. In order to implement them in IBM Intelligent Miner, we have sequentially searched for sequence rules between consecutive pairs of pages. For instance, Table 6 contains the most frequent direct sequence rules from the start_session page.

Table 6. The most frequent direct sequences of length 2 starting with start_session

Support (%)	Itemsets
45.807	start_session→ home
17.016	start_session→ program
14.516	start_session→ product
9.194	start_session→ logpost
6.774	start_session→ catalog

From Table 6 we have a more correct interpretation of the most frequent entrance pages. While in indirect rules the consequents of start_session were not necessarily adjacent, now they are so. It turns out that the most supported entrance page is home, followed by program, product, logpost and catalog. Notice that this result is also more interpretable, from a logical viewpoint.

The argument seen in Table 6 can be carried out recursively, leading to subsequent direct rules from the seen pages. All of these rules can be represented graphically as in Figure 3.

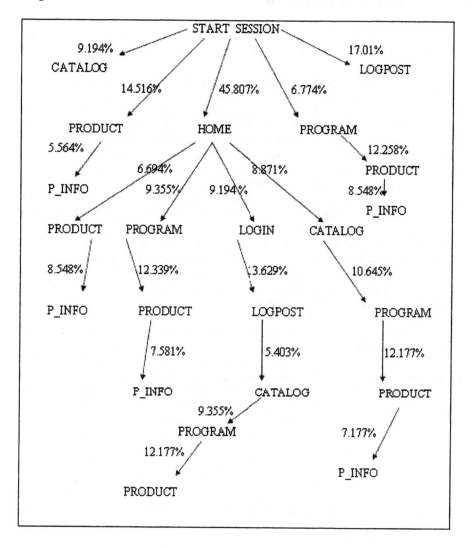

Fig. 3. Graph of the direct rules.

Figure 3 can be used to describe the most frequent navigation patterns of the visitors, as expressed by direct sequence rules. Above each link are reported the support probabilities of the corresponding rule. For instance, from Figure 3 it turns out that one of the most likely path starts from start_session, to home, than to program, than to product and, finally, to p_info.

6 Probabilistic Expert Systems

For comparison purposes, we finally present a directed graphical model, that, differently from before, is based on a probabilistic model, thereby allowing inferential results.

The main motivation to use an expert system is that association rules are simply descriptive and also a local methods. Therefore, in order to enforce their validity, a probabilistic model is needed. An expert system is a probabilistic model which can be built by means of a sequence of local models; yet, at the same time, it is a global model, and thus takes into account all interrelationships between variables.

A probabilistic expert system (see, for instance, Lauritzen, 1996, or Whittaker, 1990) is a directed graphical model in which the link between the variables is not symmetric, but rather asymmetrical. However, we signal that assuming a causal not reversible sequence among the binary variables of visit to the single pages is not fully a realistic hypothesis. In fact, since the "feedbacks" are rather frequent and the input data set does not contain information about the visit order, it is not evidently possible to assume that the causality relations are determined by the time visit order.

The expert system represented in figure 3 has been obtained on the basis of 19 models of logistic regression, one model of logistic regression for each of the 19 pages most frequented, which were acting from time to time as response variables. In each of them, the 18 remaining binary variables have been all used as explanatory variables.

For comparison purposes, we have left in the graph only the links that correspond to positive associations.

In particular, the directed graphical model has been built supposing that, if a significantly positive odds ratio had occured, this would have corresponded to the existence of a causal link from the explanatory variable at issue to the target variable. Graphically, we have represented the single causal links, so identified, by an one-way arrow which leaves from the explanatory variable and arrives at the target variable.

The model in Figure 4 gives a different representation of the most likely web clickstream paths. Differently from before, the model is based on the contingency table that is obtained from the visitor's dataset, without taking order really into account. This may be seen as a disadvantage. On the other hand, the advantage of the probabilistic expert systems is that it is based on inferential results, thus more stable with respect to the observed data. Finally, the expert system is a global model, that takes correctly into account the multivariate dependencies between variables, while the graph in Figure 3 is a local model.

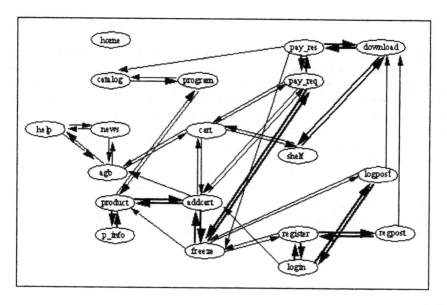

Fig. 4. Probabilistic expert system.

7 Comparison of the Methods

We have considered two classes of statistical models to model web clickstream data. It is quite difficult to choose between them. Here the situation is complicated by the fact that we have to compare local models (such as sequence rules) with global models (such as probabilistic expert systems).

For global models, such as probabilistic expert systems, statistical evaluation can proceed in terms of classical scoring methods, such as likelihood ratio scoring, AIC or BIC. Or, alternatively, by means of computationally intensive predictive evaluation, based on cross-validation and/or bootstrapping. But the real problem is how to compare them with sequence rules.

A simple and natural scoring function of a sequence rule is its support, that gives the proportion of the population to which the rule applies. Another measure of interestingness of a rule, with respect to a situation of irrelevance, is the lift of the rule itself. The lift is the ratio between the support of the confidence of the rule $A \rightarrow B$ and the support of B. Recalling the definition of the confidence index, the lift compares the observed absolute frequency of the rule with that corresponding to independence between A and B.

Ultimately, though, the assessment of an association pattern has to be judged by their utility for the objectives of the analysis at hand. In the present case-study, for instance, the informative value of the start_session $\rightarrow$ end_session rule, which in table 1 has the largest support and confidence (100%) is, for instance, null. On the other hand, the informative value of the rules that go from start_session to other pages, and from other pages to end_session can be extremely important for the design of the website.

8 Conclusions

In this paper we have presented two methodologies for the analysis of web clickstream data. The first one is based on classical association and sequence rules. We have proposed a method that calculates direct sequence rules explicitly. By means of association rules one is able to understand local associations between visited pages. Association rules are relatively easy to extract and interpret. However, it is difficult to have a global picture of what is going on.

The second methodology, on the other hand, is based on a more sophisticated statistical model, a probabilistic expert system. We have proposed a simple implementation of such models. Probabilistic expert systems are global in nature, and they thus allow an overall interpretation of the associations. On the other hand, the specification and interpretation of such models may be quite difficult.

We thus conclude that both methodologies should be considered in practical applications, and the choice accomplished on the basis of the objectives of the analysis.

References

1. BLANC E., GIUDICI P. (2002): Statistical Models for web clickstream analysis, Technical Report, Submitted.
2. BLANC E., TARANTOLA C. (2002): Dependency Networks and Bayesian Networks for Web Mining, Technical Report, Submitted.
3. CABENA P., HADJINIAN P., STADLER R., VERHEES J. and ZANASI A. (1997): Discovering Data Mining from Concept to Implementation, Prentice-Hall, New York.
4. DI SCALA L., LA ROCCA L. (2002): A Markov Model for Web Data, Technical Report, Submitted.
5. GIUDICI P. (2001): Metodi statistici per le applicazioni di Data Mining, McGraw-Hill Libri Italia, Milano.
6. HAN J., KAMBER M. (2000), Data Mining: Concepts and Tecniques, Morgan Kaufmann.
7. HAND D. J., HEIKKI M., PADHRAIC SMYTH (2001), Principles of Data Mining, MIT Press.
8. HASTIE, T., TIBSHIRANI, R., FRIEDMAN, J. (2001): The elements of statistical learning: data mining, inference and prediction, Springer-Verlag.
9. LAURITZEN S. (1996): Graphical Models, Clarendon Press, Oxford.
10. ROGNONI M., GIUDICI P., POLPETTINI P. (2002): Statistical models for the forecast of the visit sequences on web site, Technical Reports, Submitted.
11. SRIVASTAVA J., COOLEY R., DESHPANDE M. and TAN P. (2000): Web Usage Mining: Discovery and Applications of Usage Patterns from Web Data, SIGKDD Explorations, vol. I, Issue 2, 12-23.
12. WHITTAKER J. (1990): Graphical Models in Applied Multivariate Statistics, Wiley, Chichester.

Data Mining of Association Rules and the Process of Knowledge Discovery in Databases

Jochen Hipp[1], Ulrich Güntzer[2], and Gholamreza Nakhaeizadeh[1]

[1] DaimlerChrysler AG, Research & Technology, 89081 Ulm, Germany
jochen.hipp@daimlerchrysler.com
rheza.nakhaeizadeh@daimlerchrysler.com
[2] Wilhelm Schickard-Institute, University of Tübingen, 72076 Tübingen, Germany
guentzer@informatik.uni-tuebingen.de

Abstract. In this paper we deal with association rule mining in the context of a complex, interactive and iterative knowledge discovery process. After a general introduction covering the basics of association rule mining and of the knowledge discovery process in databases we draw the attention to the problematic aspects concerning the integration of both. Actually, we come to the conclusion that with regard to human involvement and interactivity the current situation is far from being satisfying. In our paper we tackle this problem on three sides: First of all there is the algorithmic complexity. Although today's algorithms efficiently prune the immense search space the achieved run times do not allow true interactivity. Nevertheless we present a rule caching schema that significantly reduces the number of mining runs. This schema helps to gain interactivity even in the presence of extreme run times of the mining algorithms. Second, today the mining data is typically stored in a relational database management system. We present an efficient integration with modern database systems which is one of the key factors in practical mining applications. Third, interesting rules must be picked from the set of generated rules. This might be quite costly because the generated rule sets normally are quite large whereas the percentage of useful rules is typically only a very small fraction. We enhance the traditional association rule mining framework in order to cope with this situation.

1 Introduction

During the second half of the eighties digital information technology completed its victory by conquering even the last niches in our modern world. Today nearly everything is "digitized". This development is not restricted to the obvious domains, like the Internet, common database applications, or electronic commerce. Even traditional domains of our everyday life increasingly depend on modern information technology. Examples are the scanner based cash desk at our supermarket, the electronic break system in our car, or the virtual trainer in our fitness center.

P. Perner (Ed.): Advances in Data Mining 2002, LNAI 2394, pp. 15–36, 2002.

As a result gathering data that mirrors our world has become fairly easy and rather inexpensive. On the one hand the obtained data collections for sure contain valuable and detailed information but on the other hand analyzing such massive datasets turned out to be much harder than expected. In brief, sizes ranging from tens of megabytes upto several terabytes forbid simply employing common analysis methods. Consequently during the last ten years specialized techniques have been developed that can be subsumed under the term data mining. The main goal behind these methods is to allow the efficient analysis of even very large datasets. With its origins in machine learning, statistics and databases, data mining has developed to a prospering and very active research field since the early nineties.

Since its introduction in [2] the task of association rule mining has received a great deal of attention. Today the generation of association rules is one of the most popular data mining methods. The idea of mining association rules originates from the analysis of market-basket data where rules like "A customer who buys products $x_1, x_2, \ldots, x_n$ will also buy product y with probability $c\%$" are generated.

Their direct applicability to business problems together with their inherent understandability – even for non data mining experts – made association rules such a popular mining method. Moreover it became clear that association rules are not restricted to dependency analysis in the context of retail applications but are successfully applicable to a wide range of business problems.

In this paper we deal with association rules in the context of a complex, interactive and iterative knowledge discovery process. In Section 2 we formally introduce association rules and give a first example. Then in Section 3 we draw the attention to the process of knowledge discovery in databases (KDD) and describe its basics. At the end of this section we finally explain the implications on association rule mining. Concerning human involvement and interactivity we come to the conclusion that today the situation is still not satisfying but there are several main starting points to cope with this problem:

First of all there is the algorithmic complexity. In brief, the number of rules grows exponentially with the number of items. Fortunately today's algorithms are able to efficiently prune this immense search space based on minimal thresholds for quality measures on the rules. We deal with the details of rule generation in Section 4.

Second, the mining data is typically stored in a relational database management system. Therefore efficient and elegant integration with modern database systems is one of the key factors in practical mining applications. The reason is that simple solutions like flat file extraction of the data quickly reach their limits in the context of massive datasets and repeated algorithms runs. A solution to this problem is given in Section 5.

Third, interesting rules must be picked from the set of generated rules. This might be quite costly because the generated rule sets normally are quite large – e.g. more than $100,000$ rules are not uncommon – and in contrast the percentage of useful rules is typically only a very small fraction. In Section 6 we enhance the traditional association rule mining framework in order to cope with this situation. In addition we present a rule caching schema that allows reducing the number of mining runs. This schema helps to gain interactivity even in the presence of extreme run times of the mining algorithms.

2   Association Rules

As mentioned, association rules are a popular mining method for dependency analysis. In this section we formally define association rules and give an illustrative example. In addition we introduce further rule quality measures that supplement the basic support-confidence framework.

2.1   Formal Definition and Example

Let $\mathcal{I} = \{x_1, \ldots, x_n\}$ be a set of distinct literals, called items. A set $X \subseteq \mathcal{I}$ with $k = |X|$ is called a k-itemset or simply an itemset. Let a database $\mathcal{D}$ be a multi-set of subsets of $\mathcal{I}$. Each $T \in \mathcal{D}$ is called a transaction.

We say that a transaction $T \in \mathcal{D}$ supports an itemset $X \subseteq \mathcal{I}$ if $X \subseteq T$ holds. Let $X, Y \subseteq \mathcal{I}$ be nonempty itemsets with $X \cap Y = \emptyset$. Then an association rule is an implication

$$X \to Y,$$

with rule body X, rule head Y, and rule confidence

$$\mathsf{conf}(X \to Y) = \frac{|\{T \in \mathcal{D} \mid X \cup Y \subseteq T\}|}{|\{T \in \mathcal{D} \mid X \subseteq T\}|}.$$

The confidence can be understood as the conditional probability $P(Y|X)$. The fraction of transactions T supporting an itemset X with respect to database $\mathcal{D}$ is called the support of X,

$$\mathsf{supp}(X) = \frac{|\{T \in \mathcal{D} \mid X \subseteq T\}|}{|\mathcal{D}|}.$$

The support of a rule $X \to Y$ is defined as

$$\mathsf{supp}(X \to Y) = \mathsf{supp}(X \cup Y).$$

In the following we want to give a simple numeric example for further illustration. In Table 1 a database $\mathcal{D}$, consisting of eight different transactions, respectively vehicles together with installed special equipments, is shown.

There are five different items, namely: AirConditioning, 2ndAirbag, Battery-TypeC, Clutch, and RadioTypeE. The support of item AirConditioning is

$$\mathsf{supp}(\mathsf{AirConditioning}) = \frac{|\{v_1, v_4, v_5\}|}{|\mathcal{D}|} = \frac{3}{8} = 37,5\%$$

Table 1. Vehicles and installed special equipment

Vehicle	Special Equipment
v_1	{AirConditioning, 2ndAirbag, BatteryTypeC}
v_2	{Clutch, RadioTypeE}
v_3	{}
v_4	{AirConditioning, BatteryTypeC}
v_5	{AirConditioning, Clutch, BatteryTypeC}
v_6	{RadioTypeE, BatteryTypeC}
v_7	{BatteryTypeC}
v_8	{2ndAirbag, BatteryTypeC}

The item BatteryTypeC has support:

$$\mathrm{supp}(\mathsf{BatteryTypeC}) = \frac{|\{v_1, v_4, v_5, v_6, v_7, v_8\}|}{|\mathcal{D}|} = \frac{6}{8} = 75\%$$

At the same time the support of the itemset {AirConditioning, BatteryTypeC} is:

$$\mathrm{supp}(\{\mathsf{AirConditioning},\ \mathsf{BatteryTypeC}\}) = \frac{|\{v_1, v_4, v_5\}|}{|\mathcal{D}|} = \frac{3}{8} = 37,5\%$$

The rule {AirConditioning} → {BatteryTypeC} then has the confidence

$$\mathrm{conf}(\{\mathsf{AirCondition.}\} \to \{\mathsf{BatteryTypeC}\}) = \frac{\mathrm{supp}(\{\mathsf{AirCondition.},\mathsf{BatteryTypeC}\})}{\mathrm{supp}(\{\mathsf{AirCondition.}\})} = 100\%$$

That is, whenever AirConditioning is installed the special battery type Battery-TypeC is implied. In contrast, the reverse of this rule has a much weaker confidence:

$$\mathrm{conf}(\{\mathsf{BatteryTypeC}\} \to \{\mathsf{AirConditioning}\}) = \frac{\mathrm{supp}(\{\mathsf{BatteryTypeC},\mathsf{AirCondition.}\})}{\mathrm{supp}((\{\mathsf{BatteryTypeC}\})} = 50\%$$

An explanation may be the following: The installation of AirConditioning relies on a strong power supply. For that reason the stronger BatteryTypeC is always installed together with AirConditioning. But AirConditioning is not the only reason to install a stronger battery. In fact, the second rule states that only in half of the cases BatteryTypeC is installed together with AirConditioning. Typically we are interested in rules with comparably high confidence values. conf = 100% is rather seldom but typically values from 80% upwards may be worth further attention.

In real-world applications the number of transactions easily reaches tens of millions or more and the number of items is between several thousands up to several hundred thousands.

2.2   Further Rule Quality Measures

In practice the described support-confidence framework turns out to be not as powerful as it seems at first glance. The reason is that association rules are based on correlations and do not necessarily imply causation. To further illustrate this point let us look at the following example:

Let $P(X)$ be the probability that a transaction T from database $\mathcal{D}$ contains the itemset X. Let $P(X, Y)$ be the probability that both X and Y are contained in $T \in \mathcal{D}$. Now let X and Y be stochastically independent:

$$P(X) \cdot P(Y) = P(X, Y).$$

Then for the confidence of the rule $X \rightarrow Y$ follows

$$\text{conf}(X \rightarrow Y) = P(Y).$$

This simple observation shows a severe shortcoming of the support-confidence framework. As soon as the itemset Y occurs comparably often in the data the rule $X \rightarrow Y$ also has a high confidence value. This suggests a dependency of Y from X although in fact both itemsets are stochastically independent. To cope with this problem additional rule quality measures have been developed.

Lift (Interest) [7,19]

$$\text{lift}(X \rightarrow Y) = \frac{\text{conf}(X \rightarrow Y)}{P(Y)} = \frac{\text{conf}(X \rightarrow Y)}{\text{supp}(Y)}$$

Lift directly addresses the above problem by expressing the deviation of the rule confidence from $P(Y)$. In the case of stochastic independence lift $= 1$ holds true. In contrast, a value higher than 1 means that the existence of X as part of a transaction "lifts" the probability for this transaction to also contain Y by factor lift. The opposite is true for lift values lower than one. lift is symmetric and therefore is an undirected measure.

Conviction [7]

$$\text{conv}(X \rightarrow Y) = \frac{P(X)P(\neg Y)}{P(X, \neg Y)}$$

Let $P(\neg Y)$ be the probability of a transaction $T \in \mathcal{D}$ with $Y \not\subseteq T$ and $P(X, \neg Y)$ the probability of drawing a transaction out of $\mathcal{D}$ that contains X but not Y. conv$(X \rightarrow Y)$ now expresses in how far X and $\neg Y$ are stochastically independent. High values for conv$(X \rightarrow Y)$ – up to ∞ where $P(X, \neg Y) = 0$ – express the conviction that this rule represents a causation. It is important to note that conv is not symmetric and therefore is a directed measure.

3   The Process of Knowledge Discovery

Practical experiences showed that discovering knowledge from huge databases affords much more than simply applying a sophisticated data mining algorithm to a predefined dataset. In fact, people from research and practice more and more understand knowledge discovery in databases (KDD) as the nontrivial process of identifying valid, novel, potentially useful, and ultimately understandable patterns in data. [10]

In this context pattern is meant in a very general way. A pattern is whatever a data mining algorithm may find in or generate from the data, e.g. a model that scores customers based on a decision tree or based on a neural network, a clustering of the data, or a set of association rules. Whereas the demand for validity, novelty, usefulness and understandability of these patterns is ultimately clear, the implications of the term "nontrivial process" might not be obvious at first glance and are worth a deeper look.

3.1   The Phases of the KDD Process

A KDD process consists of several tasks. Indeed, the actual mining, that is to say the application of a data mining algorithm to a dataset, is only one of these steps. Following the CRISP-Data Mining model [9,31] we distinguish the following tasks:

1. *Business Understanding*
   The very first step of a KDD project should be a close look from the business point of view. The goal of this phase is to gain a deeper understanding of the project objectives and further circumstances strictly from the business perspective. Finally the insights from this initial phase are to be turned into a data mining problem definition.

2. *Data Understanding*
   Based on the results from the business point of view the second step is to get familiar with the available data. The goal is to understand the attributes and the corresponding attribute values and to find out hidden semantics possibly in the data. Furthermore at this stage one should figure out what exactly the available data offers. That is to say, whether it has the potential to answer our mining questions or not, and if possible to select promising subsets of the data.

3. *Data Preparation*
   The next step is to construct the dataset where the mining algorithm is to be run on. This phase covers both syntactic aspects – format transformations for the employed mining algorithm – and semantic aspects like table, record and attribute selection. Last but not least this phase also includes deriving new attributes that contain higher information only implicitly contained in the raw data (e.g. deriving "day of the week" from "date").

4. *Modeling (or Mining)*
   In the modeling phase the actual data mining takes place. Based on the identified business goals and the assessment of the available data an appropriate mining algorithm is chosen and run on the prepared data.

5. *Evaluation*
   Evaluating the results of the mining run mainly covers three aspects. First of all, it is necessary to ensure whether everything went right from the technical point of view. Was the mining algorithms finally able to read and interpret the prepared dataset correctly? Were all designated information actually

given to the algorithm? Etc. Second, one needs to investigate whether the mining results are sound from the mining methods point of view. Some methods directly support this decision by computing certain significance measures whereas others leave this aspect completely to the analyst and his experience. Third, a key objective of the evaluation phase is to determine if all important business issues have been considered adequately.

6. *Deployment*

   After mining the data and assessing the data mining results one needs to transfer the results back into the business environment. This can be rather straight forward like preparing the results in form of a report that is understandable by business people (who of course typically are non data mining experts). Or, as the other extreme, can be quite complex like implementing a repeatable data mining process across the enterprise.

Although there is a broad number of competing process descriptions, e.g. [1, 4,8,5,9,10,30,32], all agree concerning the basic character of the KDD process: KDD is by no means a push button technology. That is to say, the analyst never walks strictly through the preprocessing tasks, mines the data, and then analyzes and deploys the results. Rather, knowledge discovery is complex, iterative and highly interactive. In each of the phases sketched above it is the analyst as a human being who decides whether to proceed to the next phase, to redo the current phase or even to step back to one of the former phases. In Figure 1 the most important of these interdependencies between the phases are indicated by arrows. The cycle around the process indicates the overall cyclic character of a KDD process.

Obviously the analysts creativity and experience have a major part in such a human centered process. Of course this nontrivial character of the KDD process pushes constraints on the employed data mining methods.

3.2   Association Rule Mining and the KDD Process

The key to human involvement is to enable analysts to interact easily with both, data and mining results. To illustrate this point further, let's look at a concrete example from dependency analysis on the features of cars: in the beginning an analyst's goal is to obtain a general "feeling" for the data. The issued mining queries are not focused but try to capture the whole available search space. As a consequence resulting rule sets are typically rather huge and overtax the analyst easily. Upto several ten thousand rules are not uncommon. In the initial phase the analyst identifies promising starting points for his further investigations. The challenge is to do this on the basis of rule sets containing a great portion of noise, trivial rules, or otherwise uninteresting associations.

After this orientation phase the analyst decides typically to take a closer look at a subset of the vehicle features. For example, he focuses on rules that contain special equipment together with information on the engine type installed. He lowers thresholds for some rule quality measures, implying a rerun of the algorithm. The results are not as expected, and the analyst suspects that the results might be more convincing if the algorithm is only applied to a subset of

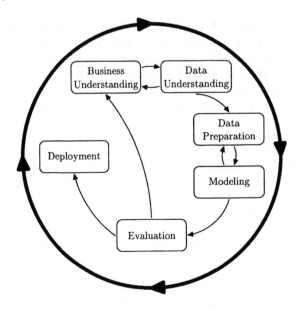

Fig. 1. The phases of the CRISP-Data Mining process

the mining data. To be more concrete, he supposes that certain dependencies may only hold true for a special model of car. Restricting the data to this model means returning to data pre-processing and implies a rerun of preparation and mining steps. Finally, it turns out that the analyst's guess was wrong. Although, he laboriously restricted the data to different models, he was not able to capture the dependency he expected. His next attempt is to take additional features of the cars investigated into consideration, etc.

After a general search phase, typically the analyst begins to focus. This second phase is characterized by trial and error and success depends largely on the skills and experience of the analyst. Still the size of the generated rule sets is problematic. Of course the search space is more and more restricted but normally this effect is outbalanced by the lowered thresholds on the rule quality measures. In addition a second problem now becomes obvious: investigating even speculative ideas often implies a rerun of the mining algorithm and possibly of data pre-processing tasks. Yet if every simple and speculative idea implies to be idle for a few minutes, then analysts will – at least in the long run – brake themselves in advance instead of trying out diligently whatever pops into their minds. So, creativity and inspiration are smothered by the annoying inefficiencies of the underlying technology. When mining for association rules on large datasets, the response times of the algorithms easily range from several minutes to hours, even with the fastest hardware and highly optimized algorithms available today, c.f. [14].

4   Rule Generation

Since the introduction of association rules in [2] a broad variety of association rule mining algorithms have been developed. The main challenge when mining association rules is the great number of rules to be considered.

4.1   Formal Problem Description

Let $\mathcal{R}$ be the number of all rules existing to a set of distinct literals $\mathcal{I}$ with $|\mathcal{I}| = n$. It follows:

$$|\mathcal{R}| = 3^n - 2^{n+1} + 1$$

Proof: For all $x, y \in \mathbb{R}$ and $n \in \mathbb{N}$ the following holds , c.f. [12, p. 57]:

$$(*) \qquad (x+y)^n = \sum_{k=0}^{n} \binom{n}{k} x^{(n-k)} y^k$$

With $x = 1$ and $y = 1$ it follows:

$$(**) \qquad 2^n = \sum_{k=0}^{n} \binom{n}{k}$$

The left side of a rule may contain up to $n - 1$ different items. With k denoting the number of items on the left side of the rule, for the right side maximally $n - k$ items are left. With that $|\mathcal{R}|$ can be expressed as follows:

$$
\begin{aligned}
|\mathcal{R}| &= \sum_{k=1}^{n-1} \sum_{l=1}^{n-k} \binom{n}{k} \binom{n-k}{l} = \sum_{k=1}^{n-1} \left(\binom{n}{k} \cdot \sum_{l=1}^{n-k} \binom{n-k}{l} \right) \\
&= \sum_{k=1}^{n-1} \left(\binom{n}{k} \cdot \left(\sum_{l=0}^{n-k} \binom{n-k}{l} - \binom{n-k}{0} \right) \right) \\
&\overset{(**)}{=} \sum_{k=1}^{n-1} \left(\binom{n}{k} \cdot (2^{n-k} - 1) \right) = \sum_{k=1}^{n-1} \left(\binom{n}{k} 2^{(n-k)} \right) - \sum_{k=1}^{n-1} \binom{n}{k} \\
&= \sum_{k=0}^{n} \left(\binom{n}{k} 2^{(n-k)} 1^k \right) - 2^n - 1 - \sum_{k=0}^{n} \binom{n}{k} + 2 \overset{(*)}{=} 3^n - 2^{n+1} + 1
\end{aligned}
$$

$\square$

In practical applications n may range from "only" about several hundred items up to several hundred thousand or even more, depending on the actual application. Therefore mining all rules obviously is infeasible. Moreover from the point of view of a person deploying association rules for analysis purposes, mining all associations would hardly make any sense. Therefore the rule set to be generated is typically restricted by minimal thresholds for the rule quality measures support and confidence, minsupp and minconf respectively.

This restriction allows [3] to split the problem into two separate parts: An itemset X is called frequent if $\mathsf{supp}(X) \geq \mathsf{minsupp}$. Once,

$$\mathcal{F} = \{X \subseteq \mathcal{I} \mid \mathsf{supp}(X) \geq \mathsf{minsupp}\},$$

the set of all frequent itemsets together with the corresponding support values is known, deriving the desired association rules is straight forward: For every $X \in \mathcal{F}$ one has to check the confidence of all rules

$$X \setminus Y \to Y$$

with $\emptyset \neq Y \subsetneq X$.

The so called downward closure property of itemset support ensures that we actually can compute all necessary confidence values, c.f. [3]. This property states that all subsets of a frequent itemset must also be frequent. So if X is frequent we also know the support of all $X \setminus Y$ with $\emptyset \neq Y \subsetneq X$.

What remains to be done before rule generation is to determine $\mathcal{F}$, the set of all frequent itemsets. Unfortunately for obvious reason we are not able to look at all subsets of $\mathcal{I}$: A linearly growing $n = |\mathcal{I}|$ of course still implies an exponential growing number of subsets to be taken into consideration.

4.2   The Generation of Frequent Itemsets

In the beginning of the mining run each itemset $X \subseteq \mathcal{I}$ is potentially frequent. In other words the initial search space consists of the power set of $\mathcal{I}$ without the empty set, $\mathcal{P}(\mathcal{I}) \setminus \emptyset$. Therefore even for rather small $|\mathcal{I}|$ the search space easily exceeds all limits. For the set of items $\mathcal{I} = \{a, b, c, d, e\}$ this search space is shown in Figure 2.

In order to avoid traversing the whole search space modern association mining algorithms employ a candidate generation and test approach. The idea is to generate an easy to survey set of potential frequent itemsets, a set of so called candidates. Then the support values of these candidates are determined based on the database $\mathcal{D}$. Candidate generation always considers all information on frequency and infrequency of already investigated candidates. In brief the common strategy is as follows: from the downward closure property of itemset support we know that all subsets of a frequent itemset must also be frequent. This allows us to immediately prune those candidates as infrequent from the search space that have at least one infrequent subset. After candidate generation the designated candidates are counted based on the database and the algorithm proceeds to the next iteration. The whole process stops as soon as there are no more potentially frequent itemsets that have not been considered as candidates.

In Figure 2 the thick border separates the frequent itemsets in the upper part from the infrequent itemsets in the lower part for a hypothetical support threshold minsupp. The existence of such a border is guaranteed by the downward closure property of itemset support. Clearly, the proposed stepwise traversal of the search space should start at the top with all or part of the frequent 1-itemsets

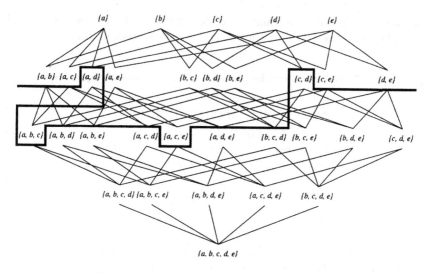

Fig. 2. The Search Space for $\mathcal{I} = \{a, b, c, d, e\}$

as candidates. Then the algorithm should descend to the lower levels. This can be done by breadth-first search or depth-first search. The border is a natural barrier where the step-wise search space traversal stops. From the itemsets below the border only the itemsets immediately at the border may be considered as candidates. Looking at these itemsets is necessary to exactly identify the course of the border.

There are two common approaches to actually determine the support of the candidates. The first approach is to directly count sets of candidates. For each candidate a counter is set up and the algorithm then passes over the complete database of transactions. Whenever a transactions contains one of the candidates its counter is incremented. Efficiently looking up candidates in transactions requires specialized data structures, e.g. hashtrees or prefix trees, c.f. [3,6].

Alternatively the support values of candidates can be determined indirectly by set intersections. For that purpose so called transaction sets are employed. The transaction set X.tids of an itemset X is defined as the set of all transactions this itemset is contained in:

$$X.\text{tids} = \{T \in \mathcal{D} \mid X \subseteq T\}.$$

For the support follows

$$\text{supp}(X) = \frac{|X.\text{tids}|}{|\mathcal{D}|}.$$

Determining the transaction sets for the frequent 1-itemsets is straight forward. It simply requires to transform the database from so called horizontal layout to vertical layout. We initialize an empty list to hold the transaction set for each item. Then we pass over all transactions and for each item in the current transaction we add a unique transaction identifier to its transaction set. For the example database from Table 1 the vertical layout is given in Table 2

Table 2. Vertical layout for vhicles and installed special equipment

Special Equipment	Vehicles
AirConditioning	$\{v_1, v_4, v_5\}$
2ndAirbag	$\{v_1, v_8\}$
BatteryTypeC	$\{v_1, v_4, v_5, v_6, v_7, v_8\}$
Clutch	$\{v_2, v_5\}$
RadioTypeE	$\{v_6\}$

The transaction sets of the n-itemsets with $n > 1$ are determined on the fly by set intersections. For each itemset Z with $Z = X \cup Y$ holds

$$Z.\text{tids} = X.\text{tids} \cap Y.\text{tids}.$$

Of course this implies that during search space traversal we need to ensure that we always have the necessary transaction sets at our hands, that is to say in main memory.

To give an example lets look at the itemset $\{\text{AirConditioning}, \text{BatteryTypeC}\}$. The transaction set of this itemset can be determined based on the transaction sets of the corresponding 1-itemsets:

$$\{\text{AirCondition.}, \text{BatteryTypeC}\}.\text{tids} = \{\text{AirCondition.}\}.\text{tids} \cap \{\text{BatteryTypeC}\}.\text{tids}$$
$$= \{v_1, v_4, v_5\} \cap \{v_1, v_4, v_5, v_6, v_7, v_8\}$$
$$= \{v_1, v_4, v_5\}$$

4.3 Algorithms

The framework for frequent itemset generation from above leaves room for several algorithmic instantiations. The most wide-spread of these algorithms is Apriori from [3]. Its pseudocode is given in Figure 3. Apriori implements the above step-wise search space traversel as a breadth-first search together with counting the candidates directly. In the beginning the set of all frequent 1-itemsets, $\mathcal{F}_1$, is determined by setting up a counter for each $x \in \mathcal{I}$ and passing over the database. Then each following level of the search space is processed separately in two phases. First of all the candidate set is generated based on the results from the previous level. All itemsets $C \in \mathcal{P}(\mathcal{I})$, $|C| = \text{level}$, for which all subsets of size $\text{level} - 1$ are frequent,

$$\forall S \subsetneq C, |S| = \text{level-1} : S \in \mathcal{F}_{\text{level}-1},$$

are included in the candidate set $\mathcal{C}_{\text{level}}$. Second, the support values of all candidates in $\mathcal{C}_{\text{level}}$ are determined in a single pass over the database. This procedure is

```
1)    𝓕₁ = {frequent 1-itemsets}
2)    for(level = 2; 𝓕ₗₑᵥₑₗ₋₁ ≠ ∅; ++level)
3)    {
4)        𝓒ₗₑᵥₑₗ = generate_candidates(𝓕ₗₑᵥₑₗ₋₁);
5)        forall transactions T ∈ 𝒟
6)        {
7)            forall C ⊆ T
8)            {
9)                if C ∈ 𝓒ₗₑᵥₑₗ then
10)                   ++C.count
11)           }
12)       }
13)   }
```

Fig. 3. Pseudocode of the Apriori algorithm [3]

repeated until no more candidates to count are generated. In other words, Apriori starts with determining all frequent 2-itemsets, proceeds with all frequent 3-itemsets etc and stops as soon as it has reached a level that is completely below the border from Figure 2.

Most other algorithms are variations of the Apriori principle. For instance Partition [26] combines the breadth-first search of Apriori with determining the support values of the candidates indirectly by set intersections. In order to be able to keep all necessary transaction sets comfortably in main memory the database typically needs to be partitioned. The algorithm DIC [6] enhances Apriori by relaxing the strict separation between candidate generation and counting the candidates. Already during passing over the transactions new candidates are generated and added to the set of candidates on the fly. This helps to significantly reduce the total number of the expensive passes over the database. Eclat [33] combines a depth-first search strategy with intersections of transaction sets. Due to depth-first search it is no longer guaranteed that all necessary information for pruning candidates based on infrequent subsets is always available. Accordingly Eclat has to live with larger candidate sets. Hybrid [15] employs a special depth-first search strategy that does not have this limitation and moreover profits from switching between breadth-first search and depth-first search during lattice traversal.

Figure 4 shows a performance benchmark covering several state of the art mining algorithms. The experiments were run on a PentiumIII clocked at 500Mhz. The algorithms were implemented in C++ and have proven their efficiency in several projects, c.f. [16,17,31]. On the logarithmically scaled x-axis the threshold minsupp is lowered from 2% down to 0.125%. On the also logarithmically scaled y-axis we find the corresponding time for frequent pattern generation. The employed dataset is a well known benchmark dataset first introduced in [3]. Its average transaction size is 10, average frequent pattern size 4, and it contains a total number of 1 million transactions. Obviously for none of

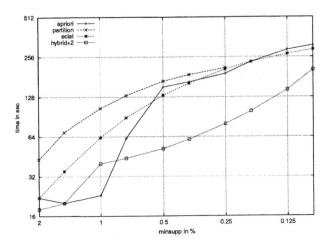

Fig. 4. Performance benchmark

the mining algorithms the achieved runtime – and actually 1 million transactions is still a moderate database size –would allow true interactivity in an iterative KDD process as introduced in Section 3. On larger databases and with lower minsupp values easily run times upto hours are reached.

5   Integration with Relational Database Systems

In Section 3 we learned that data mining – running the mining algorithm – is only one of the steps in a KDD process. In this context it becomes clear that algorithmic details are important but of course the integration of the mining algorithm with the other KDD phases must also be considered. Interactivity tremendously suffers when proceeding from one KDD phase to next is not smooth but implies annoying user interference [13].

5.1   Common Situation

Flat files or even binary encoded datasets are common in research and development environments but we rarely found them in business units. So, today in real-world applications we can expect the data to reside in a database system. For the mining algorithms this implies that a proper integration with relational database systems is one of the key features.

The natural way to store transactions as they were introduced in Section 2 in a relational table is in (id, item)-tuple form, c.f. Table 3. Each transaction (vehicle) is represented by one or more rows in the table.

But of course a database will typically not be restricted to such "transactional data". For instance in our example there will also be tables that hold attributes

Table 3. Relational representation of transaction data

VehicleId	SpecialEquipment
v_1	AirConditioning
v_1	2ndAirbag
v_1	BatteryTypeC
v_2	Clutch
v_2	RadioTypeE
v_4	AirConditioning
v_4	BatteryTypeC
v_5	AirConditioning
v_5	Clutch
v_5	BatteryTypeC
⋮	⋮

of vehicles like ModelType, EngineType, ProductionDate etc. Typically these attributes will be stored in a separate table where each vehicle is represented by exactly one row, c.f Table 4

Table 4. Vehicles together with further attributes

VehicleId	ModelType	EngineType	ProductionDate	...
⋮	⋮	⋮	⋮	⋮
v_1	W202	D	Feb 24 2002	...
v_2	W202	P	Feb 25 2002	...
v_3	W220	P	Mar 12 2002	...
v_4	W220	D	Mar 12 2002	...
v_5	W220	D	Mar 17 2002	...
⋮	⋮	⋮	⋮	⋮

Furthermore in a database like the one in our example there is probably not only a single entity like "vehicle" but also other entities representing e.g. engine model, production plant, warranty claim etc. Of course the algorithms should be able to also consider these other entities.

5.2   Technical Aspects and Implementation

As we saw in Section 4 association rule algorithms expect the data prepared as transactions. Generating such transactions from a database may require joining information pieces from all over the database. Of course it is the best to leave this task in the hands of the database system. An appropriate join statement then would collect all attributes and temporarily output them in a denormalized table. Due to the fact that not each object must be present in all of the tables an outer join is needed. An example for such a join query that generates transactions for the vehicles produced in the year 2002 from the tables vehicles and special_equipment is given in Figure 5, where the tables from Table 3 and

```
select      VehicleId, ModelType, EngineType, SpecialEquipment
from        vehicles outer join special_equipment on
            vehicles.VehicleId = special_equipment.VehicleId
where       year(vehicles.ProductionDate) = 2002
order by    vehicles.VehicleId
```

Fig. 5. Example query

Table 4 are joined. Exemplarily the resulting temporary table is shown in Table 5. Of course this table contains a lot of redundant information. Fortunately this denormalized table is temporary and we need read access only.

Table 5. Example for a temporal denormalized table

VehicleId	ModelType	EngineType	SpecialEquipment	...
⋮	⋮	⋮	⋮	⋮
v1	W202	D	AirConditioning	...
v1	W202	D	2ndAirbag	...
v1	W202	D	BatteryTypeC	...
v2	W202	P	Clutch	...
v2	W202	P	RadioTypeE	...
v3	W220	P	[NULL]	...
v4	W220	D	AirConditioning	...
v4	W220	D	BatteryTypeC	...
v5	W220	D	AirConditioning	...
v5	W220	D	Clutch	...
v5	W220	D	BatteryTypeC	...
⋮	⋮	⋮	⋮	⋮

By sorting on VehicleId we ensure that each vehicle is described by consecutive rows. To derive the desired transactions we simply pass through all rows. Whenever the key VehicleId changes we know that a new transaction starts. Otherwise we add all attributes of the row under investigation to the current transaction. It is also important to note that due to the redundancy in the table we must beware of duplicate attributes.

Each collected transaction is immediately stored in a binary cache on the file system. For that purpose the strings representing the attribute values are mapped to integers. The attribute values are enriched with the corresponding attribute name because otherwise they might easily cause ambiguities, think e.g. of color "red". So we finally obtain a dictionary that maps integers one to one onto strings and a compact binary file containing the actual transactions.

Algorithms that make several passes over the database, e.g. Apriori, greatly benefit from caching the transactions.

6 Further Integration with the KDD Process

In the previous section we treated the integration of the association mining algorithms concerning data access. In other words we showed the integration aspects from the input point of view. Now we turn over to the output side. We cover how to appropriately arrange and store the association mining results in the context of an embracing KDD process, c.f. [17].

6.1 Basic Idea

In Section 4 we learned that even the most efficient association mining algorithms still have run times of at least several minutes upto hours depending on the mining data. If we remember the KDD process exemplarily described in Section 3 it becomes clear that even interruptions of the analysts work of a single minute are already problematic.

Some authors tackle this problem by pushing constraints on the result set into the mining algorithm [22,24,25,29]. Actually the performance improves but the run times are still far from allowing true interactivity. Furthermore the constraint result set will probably answer fewer of the analysts questions and therefore will provoke additional further mining runs.

The solution that we propose is to do exactly the opposite: we broaden the result set, c.f. [17]. Instead of restricting we suggest to add everything that might make sense to the mining data and then let the mining algorithm generate all rules based on relatively low thresholds for the rule quality measures. Of course under these conditions rule generation will take its time. But what we must not forget is that even when constraining the result set as much possible we also will not gain true interactivity. So why not deliberately accepting an interruption but then proceed with interactively investigating a comprehensive rule set without any or at least very few further interruptions?

What is presumed in such a scenario is a cache to efficiently store the generated rules. Once the cache is filled by running the mining algorithm answering mining queries means retrieving the appropriate rules from the cache instead of mining them from the data. Accessing a properly implemented cache only takes seconds as shown in [17]. Of course the number of generated and stored rules will be overwhelming and the result set will probably be full of noise, trivial rules or otherwise uninteresting associations. Therefore highly sophisticated access to the cache is crucial in order not to overtax the analyst.

6.2   Enhancing the Association Mining Framework

Access to the rule cache depends on the actual mining scenario and the concrete mining questions of the analyst. It therefore must be as flexible as possible in order to be useful for a wide range of mining problems.

In Section 2 we treated items as atomic literals. This is the common way to look at items in the context of association rule mining. We found that although items are literals from the rule generation point of view, items indeed normally have structure and moreover rule retrieval could greatly benefit from exploiting this additional information.

The first step we do is breaking up the atomic items. For example items in a supermarket have prices and costs associated. Accordingly production dates, manufacturers etc are assigned to parts of vehicles. These attributes may be incorporated into the mining run by quantitative association rules [28] or generalized association rules [18,27], but typically this is not sufficient from the rule retrieval point of view.

We extent the basic framework of association mining as follows: Let $\mathcal{I} \subseteq \mathbb{N} \times \mathbb{A}_1 \times \cdots \times \mathbb{A}_m$ be the universe of items. Each item is uniquely identified by an ID $id \in \mathbb{N}$ and described by further attributes $a_1, \ldots a_m \in \mathbb{A}_1 \times \ldots \times \mathbb{A}_m$. Attributes can be from any desired domain $\mathbb{A}_n$, e.g. prices, costs, dates or other application dependent information. Also we treat the name of an item as an attached attribute. Based on this extension a set of rules is defined as $\mathcal{R} \subseteq \mathcal{P}(\mathcal{I}) \times \mathcal{P}(\mathcal{I}) \times \mathbb{R} \times \cdots \times \mathbb{R}$. As usually, in addition to the assumption and the consequence (subsets of the power set of $\mathcal{I}$), each rule is rated by a constant number of different and real valued quality measures. Adding attributes to the items in such a way does not affect the mining procedure but nevertheless introduces a new means to formulate practically important mining queries.

6.3   Rule Retrieval

In this paper we would like to describe a simple mining query language that demonstrates the potentials of our approach. Our language is very useful on its own but can also be integrated into universal environments as described in [11, 20,21,23].

Each query consists of the key word SelectRulesFrom followed by the name of the rule cache to be accessed. In the following where-clause restrictions on the rules to be retrieved are given. The basic query simply restricts the result set by thresholds on rule quality measures. For example, we may want the system to return all rules from the cache rulecache that have **confidence above 85%** and **lift of at least 15**.

```
SelectRulesFrom rulecache
Where confidence > 0.85 and lift >= 15;
```

In order to deal with thresholds on the rules relative to the actual values reached in a rule set we introduce aggregate functions on rule quality measures. The following query returns rules having rather low support and at the same time quite high confidence compared to all other rules in the cache. min(supp) denotes the minimum support value of all rules in the rule cache and max(conf) the maximum confidence respectively.

```
SelectRulesFrom rulecache
supp < 1.1 * min(supp) and conf > 0.9 * max(conf);
```

Next, we want to specify rules based on certain items. For that purpose we introduce the keywords assumption and consequent to address the items in the body and respectively the head of the rules. The following query retrieves rules containing a certain item in the rule consequent.

```
SelectRulesFrom rulecache
Where '2ndAirbag' in consequent and conf > 0.85;
```

While we do not see the need for explicit $\exists$ and $\forall$ quantifiers on sets of rules, having these on the itemsets is quite useful. In conjunction with the attributes linked to items, powerful queries become possible. For example we could select all rules that have support higher than 5%, confidence higher than 95%, and that "explain" at least one special equipment which incurs costs above a certain threshold. In the following x.attributename gives the value of attribute attributename for item x:

```
SelectRulesFrom rulecache
Where supp > 0.05 and conf > 0.95
and exists x in consequence (x.type = 'spec equip'
and x.costs > 1000);
```

A more complex and also very useful query is to find all rules with nothing but special equipment in the consequence originating from a manufacturer who also manufactures at least one special equipment from the rule assumption.

```
SelectRulesFrom rulecache
Where forall x in consequence (x.type = 'spec equip'
and exists y in assumption (y.type = 'spec equip' and
x.manu = y.manu));
```

The quantifiers and attributes on the items and the aggregate functions on the rules are both intuitive to use and flexible. The examples above give a first impression of their potentials.

7   Summary

In this paper we dealt with association rule mining in the context of a complex, interactive and iterative knowledge discovery process. We introduced the basics of association rules and of the algorithmic aspects of association rule mining.

Furthermore we covered the fundamentals of the process of knowledge discovery in databases.

From both we learned that with regard to human involvement and interactivity the current situation is far from being satisfying. We worked out the basic problem and than tackled it on three sides:

First of all there is the algorithmic complexity. We demonstrated that today's state of the art algorithms offer impressive performance with regard to the immense search space they need to deal with. Anyway we came to the conclusion that this is still not enough to allow true interactivity in a human centered KDD process. Nevertheless we present a rule caching schema that significantly reduces the number of mining runs. This schema helps to gain interactivity even in the presence of extreme run times of the mining algorithms. Accessing a properly implemented cache only takes seconds.

Second, we pointed out that the integration of the mining algorithm with the other KDD phases is also a crucial aspect. Interactivity tremendously suffers when proceeding from one KDD phase to next is not smooth but implies annoying user interference. For that purpose we present an efficient integration of association rule mining algorithms with modern database systems.

Third, interesting rules must be picked by the data mining analyst from the set of generated rules. This might be quite costly because the generated rule sets normally are quite large – e.g. more than 100, 000 rules are not uncommon – whereas the percentage of useful rules is typically only a very small fraction. We enhanced the traditional association rule mining framework by giving structure to the items. Adding attributes to the items as proposed does not affect the mining procedure but introduces a new means to formulate practically important mining queries.

References

1. P. Adriaans and D. Zantinge. *Data Mining*. Addison-Wesley, Harlow, England, 1996.
2. R. Agrawal, T. Imielinski, and A. Swami. Mining association rules between sets of items in large databases. In *Proceedings of the ACM SIGMOD International Conference on Management of Data (ACM SIGMOD '93)*, pages 207–216, Washington, USA, May 1993.
3. R. Agrawal and R. Srikant. Fast algorithms for mining association rules. In *Proceedings of the 20th International Conference on Very Large Databases (VLDB '94)*, Santiago, Chile, June 1994.
4. T. Barth. Guidelines for the data mining process. Technical report, University of Stuttgart, Stuttgart, Germany, 1998. ESPRIT Project Number 22700.
5. R. J. Brachman and T. Anand. The process of knowledge discovery in databases: A human centered approach. In U. M. Fayyad, G. Piatetsky-Shapiro, P. Smyth, and R. Uthurusamy, editors, *Advances in Knowledge Discovery and Data Mining*, chapter 2, pages 37–57. AAAI/MIT Press, 1996.
6. S. Brin, R. Motwani, and C. Silverstein. Beyond market baskets: Generalizing association rules to correlations. In *Proceedings of the ACM SIGMOD International Conference on Management of Data (ACM SIGMOD '97)*, pages 265–276, 1997.

7. S. Brin, R. Motwani, J. D. Ullman, and S. Tsur. Dynamic itemset counting and implication rules for market basket data. In *Proceedings of the ACM SIGMOD International Conference on Management of Data (ACM SIGMOD '97)*, pages 265–276, 1997.

8. C. E. Brodley and P. Smyth. The process of applying machine learning algorithms. In *Presented at Workshop on Applying Machine Learning in Practice, 12th International Machine Learning Conference (IMLC 95)*, Tahoe City, CA, 1995.

9. P. Chapman, J. Clinton, R. Kerber, T. Khabaza, T. Reinartz, C. Shearer, and R. Wirth. CRISP-DM 1.0. http://www.crisp-dm.org/, 2000.

10. U. Fayyad, G. Piatetsky-Shapiro, and P. Smyth. The KDD process for extracting useful knowledge from volumes of data. *Communications of the ACM*, 39(11):27–34, November 1996.

11. J. Han, Y. Fu, W. Wang, K. Koperski, and O. Zaiane. DMQL: A data mining query language for relational databases. In *Proceedings of the 1996 SIGMOD'96 Workshop on Research Issues on Data Mining and Knowledge Discovery (DMKD '96)*, Montreal, Canada, June 1996.

12. H. Heuser. *Lehrbuch der Analysis*. B. G. Teubner Verlag, Stuttgart, 8 edition, 1990.

13. J. Hipp, U. Güntzer, and U. Grimmer. Integrating association rule mining algorithms with relational database systems. In *Proceedings of the 3rd International Conference on Enterprise Information Systems (ICEIS 2001)*, pages 130–137, Setúbal, Portugal, July 7-10 2001.

14. J. Hipp, U. Güntzer, and G. Nakhaeizadeh. Algorithms for association rule mining – a general survey and comparison. *SIGKDD Explorations*, 2(1):58–64, July 2000.

15. J. Hipp, U. Güntzer, and G. Nakhaeizadeh. Mining association rules: Deriving a superior algorithm by analysing today's approaches. In *Proceedings of the 4th European Symposium on Principles of Data Mining and Knowledge Discovery (PKDD '00)*, pages 159–168, Lyon, France, September 13-16 2000.

16. J. Hipp and G. Lindner. Analysing warranty claims of automobiles. an application description following the CRISP-DM data mining process. In *Proceedings of 5th International Computer Science Conference (ICSC '99)*, pages 31–40, Hong Kong, China, December 13-15 1999.

17. J. Hipp, C. Mangold, U. Güntzer, and G. Nakhaeizadeh. Efficient rule retrieval and postponed restrict operations for association rule mining. In *Proceedings of the Sixth Pacific-Asia Conference on Knowledge Discovery and Data Mining (PAKDD'02)*, May 6-8 2002.

18. J. Hipp, A. Myka, R. Wirth, and U. Güntzer. A new algorithm for faster mining of generalized association rules. In *Proceedings of the 2nd European Symposium on Principles of Data Mining and Knowledge Discovery (PKDD '98)*, pages 74–82, Nantes, France, Sept. 23–26 1998.

19. IBM. *Intelligent Miner Handbook*, 1999.

20. T. Imielinski, A. Virmani, and A. Abdulghani. Data mining: Application programming interface and query language for database mining. In *Proceedings of the 2nd International Conference on Knowledge Discovery in Databases and Data Mining (KDD '96)*, pages 256–262, Portland, Oregon, USA, August 1996.

21. T. Imielinski, A. Virmani, and A. Abdulghani. DMajor - application programming interface for database mining. *Data Mining and Knowledge Discovery*, 3(4):347–372, December 1999.

22. L. Lakshmanan, R. Ng, J. Han, and A. Pang. Optimization of constrained frequent set queries: 2-var constraints. In *3rd SIGMOD'98 Workshop on Research Issues in Data Mining and Knowledge Discovery (DMKD)*, pages 157–168, Seattle, WA, June 1998.

23. R. Meo, G. Psaila, and S. Ceri. A new sql-like operator for mining association rules. In *Proceedings of the 22nd International Conference on Very Large Databases (VLDB '96)*, Mumbai (Bombay), India, September 1996.

24. R. Ng, L. S. Lakshmanan, J. Han, and T. Mah. Exploratory mining via constrained frequent set queries. In *Proceedings of the 1999 ACM-SIGMOD International Conference on Management of Data (SIGMOD '99)*, pages 556–558, Philadelphia, PA, USA, June 1999.

25. R. Ng, L. S. Lakshmanan, J. Han, and A. Pang. Exploratory mining and pruning optimizations of constrained associations rules. In *Proceedings of 1998 ACM SIG-MOD International Conference on Management of Data (SIGMOD '98)*, Seattle, Washington, USA, June 1998.

26. A. Savasere, E. Omiecinski, and S. Navathe. An efficient algorithm for mining association rules in large databases. In *Proceedings of the 21st Conference on Very Large Databases (VLDB '95)*, pages 432–444, Zürich, Switzerland, September 1995.

27. R. Srikant and R. Agrawal. Mining generalized association rules. In *Proceedings of the 21st Conference on Very Large Databases (VLDB '95)*, Zürich, Switzerland, September 1995.

28. R. Srikant and R. Agrawal. Mining quantitative association rules in large relational tables. In *Proceedings of the 1996 ACM SIGMOD Conference on Management of Data*, Montreal, Canada, June 1996.

29. R. Srikant, Q. Vu, and R. Agrawal. Mining association rules with item constraints. In *Proceedings of the 3rd International Conference on KDD and Data Mining (KDD '97)*, Newport Beach, California, August 1997.

30. G. J. Williams and Z. Huang. Modelling the kdd process. Technical report, CSIRO Division of Information Technology, GPO Box 664 Canberra ACT 2601 Australia, Februar 1996.

31. R. Wirth, M. Borth, and J. Hipp. When distribution is part of the semantics: A new problem class for distributed knowledge discovery. In *Proceedings of the PKDD 2001 Workshop on Ubiquitous Data Mining for Mobile and Distributed Environments*, pages 56–64, Freiburg, Germany, September 3-7 2001.

32. R. Wirth and J. Hipp. CRISP-DM: Towards a standard process modell for data mining. In *Proceedings of the 4th International Conference on the Practical Applications of Knowledge Discovery and Data Mining*, pages 29–39, Manchester, UK, April 2000.

33. M. J. Zaki, S. Parthasarathy, M. Ogihara, and W. Li. New algorithms for fast discovery of association rules. In *Proceedings of the 3rd International Conference on KDD and Data Mining (KDD '97)*, Newport Beach, California, August 1997.

Intelligent E-marketing with Web Mining, Personalization, and User-Adpated Interfaces

Petra Perner and G. Fiss

Institute of Computer Vision and Applied Computer Sciences
Arno-Nitzsche-Str. 45, 04277 Leipzig
ibaiperner@aol.com http://www.ibai-research.de

Abstract. For many people the special attraction of E-commerce is linked to the idea of being able to choose and order products and services directly on-line from home. However, this is only one aspect of the new on-line sales model. As in real sales processes competent counselling, in accordance with the customer's necessities, and also after-sales assistance by help of the web play an important part for the customer faith. This requires precise knowledge of the customer's preferences who, however, in general does not like lengthy questioning and the use of other communication routes. Holders of E-shops have thus to gather the consumer's desires and preferences from his interactions and the data resulting from the sales process, which requires a profound data analysis. In this paper we describe what kind of data can be acquired in an e-shop and how these data can be used to improve advertisement, marketing and selling. We describe what kind of data mining methods are necessary and how they can be applied to the data.

Keywords. E-commerce, Data Mining, User Profiling, Clickstream analysis, Recommendation, User-Adapted Interfaces

1 Introduction

For many people the special attraction of E-commerce is linked to the idea of being able to choose and order products and services directly on-line from home. However, this is only one aspect of the new on-line sales model. As in real sales processes competent counselling, in accordance with the customer's necessities, and also after-sales assistance by help of the web play an important part for the customer faith. This requires precise knowledge of the customer's preferences who, however, in general does not like lengthy questioning and the use of other communication routes. Holders of E-shops have thus to gather the consumer's desires and preferences from his interactions and the data resulting from the sales process, which requires a profound data analysis. This knowledge has then to be converted into an intelligent and, if possible, entertaining presentation of the information wanted by the customer, where multimedia means of expression are used, and without overstraining or understraining him. Only in this way can he be motivated to continue the dialogue. As the capacities, preferences and interests of the customers vary considerably in this field of application, intelligent user guidance is indispensable.

P. Perner (Ed.): Advances in Data Mining 2002, LNAI 2394, pp. 37–52, 2002.
© Springer-Verlag Berlin Heidelberg 2002

In Section 2 of this paper we describe the main problem that are concerned with E-Marketing and Selling and why data mining and user modeling is important. The basic data that can be automatically accessed from a website are describe in Section 3. In Section 4 we give a brief overview about the basic data mining methods and indicate how they can be used for marketing and selling. In Section 5 we describe our idea for intelligent e-marketing with data mining and user-adapted interfaces. Finally we give conclusions in Section 6.

2 E-marketing/Selling

In order to do e-marketing, it is necessary to know about traditional marketing, computing sciences and also about analytical methods.

E-marketing is the concentration of all efforts in the sense of adapting and developing marketing strategies into the web environment. E-marketing involves all stages of work regarding a web site, such as the conception, the project itself, the adaptation of the content, the development, the maintenance, the analytic measuring and the advertisement. One of the most serious misunderstandings is to face the web as a simple extension of marketing campaigns of the company, or "a cheap" institutional propaganda. When launching a business on the Internet, whether it is an institutional site or a site for online shopping/electronic trade, it is necessary to have in mind that this means dealing with media, with very peculiar characteristics.

E-Business can be any site with commercial purposes that is on the internet, regardless of the characteristics of the site. A classification of these activities according to different objectives leads to four basic forms of the usage of the internet for business [1]:

• Online promotion
• Online Shopping
• Online Service and
• Online Collaboration.

The aim of online promotion is to bring an advertisement message which is targeted to specific customer group quickly and cost-effective to this group. Online-shopping is the selling of products or services via the internet. The basic requirements for an on-line shop are at least a product catalogue and a safe and error-tolerant transaction line for ordering and paying the products and services. Online-service means to provide services via the internet. These services can be free or the user has to pay a fee for it. The important advantage is that these services can be accessed from everywhere in the world at any time. With online-collaboration are named all strategies where users are enabled to get into contact with other users. Very popular are user forums (moderated and free ones). The other very common way are chat rooms. The aim of online collaboration is to transport a special image to the target group, that is not creatable through classic advertisement.

For a successful web presence it is useful to combine these different models. An online shop will also do some promotion of products via e-mail or provide services to the customer which will help to keep the customer. Successful web presentations are a full integrated part of the hole marketing and communications strategy, requiring on the general principles of e-marketing:

- Interactive and Flexible
- Informative
- Instantaneous
- Measurable
- Affordable and
- Intuitive navigation

It is important to set up the e-business model in such a way that it uses the 6 principles of e-marketing on the one hand and on the other hand meets the customer's or user's personal requirements for services, products and information. This requires to know and to understand the behavior, needs and expectations of the target group.

Apart from traditional marketing based on market research e-marketing can and should use the data given by users while they are navigating through the web site. Focusing on permission marketing where the user allows you to use his data for further communication, you are able to build up a long-lasting customer relationship. By this you can see customer data as the real treasure. To use it requires a good e-business model, data warehousing and especially data mining techniques.

A good user model is the basis for all activities. However, such customer groups are not static, they will chance over time. The internet is a fast medium. The interest of customer groups will change quickly. Customers will move away from one provider to another one. Besides that arises the question: Are your services or products appropriate to get sold via the internet? What should your web pages look like? What technological facilities has the customer who is visiting your web site?

To keep the customer's attention for your web presence requires to build up a strong customer relationship and to offer services which attract the customer to visit the web site frequently and purchase products and services. The need to develop specific marketing strategies for the internet implies that some traditional principles are adapted, or even reinvented. An online-shop offers all the incriedents (for e.g. marketing/selling data, server data, web meta data) to solve and to automate these tasks successfully (see Fig. 1). While a customer is visiting a web site he leaves a trace of data which can be used to understand the customers needs, desires and demands as well as to improve your web presence.

3 The Data

In an e-commerce site are available data across the merchandising data, marketing data, server data, and web meta data. These data can be used for data mining to better understand the marketing and selling processes, the site organization and the server itself (see Fig. 1).

There are different types of data: user entry data, server and cookie logs, web documents and web meta data.

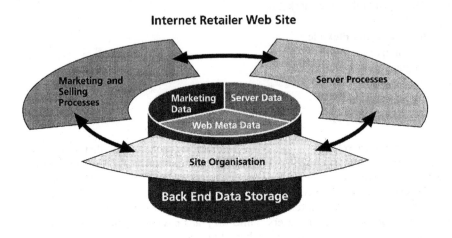

Fig. 1. Internet Retailer Web Site and available Data

3.1 Server and Cookie Data

Web server logs (see Fig. 2) are automatically generated by the server when a user is visiting an URL at a site. In a server log are registered the IP address of the visitor, the time when he is entering the website, the time duration he is visiting the requested URL and the URL he is visiting. From these information can be generated the path the user is going on this website [2]. Web server logs are important information in order to discover the behavior of the user at the website. However, the IP address stored in the server log does not always lead to the particular user. The address might have been changed by the proxy server and the heuristic used for the identification of a user session does not always hold. Therefore cookie logs might be more preferable.

Cookies are short text files that are generated by the server on the client site while his browser is visiting the website. Cookies allow to set a special identification number or code for a particular user. Each time a user is visiting the website he can be identified by this identification code. However to set a cookie requires that the user has given permission for that which is not always the case. Therefore only the combination of server logs and cookie log will be a good basis for data mining.

In the example given in Figure 2 a typical server log file is shown. Table 1 shows the code for the URL. In Table 2 is shown the path the user is taking on this website. The user has been visiting the website 4 times. A user session is considered to be closed when the user is not taking a new action within 20 minutes. This is a rule of thumb that might not always be true. Since in our example the time duration between the first user access starting at 1: 54 and the second one at 2:24 is longer than 20 minutes we consider the first access and the second access as two sessions. However, it might be that the user was staying on this website for more than 20 minutes since he was not entering the website by the main page.

hs2-210.handshake.de - - [01/Sep/1999:00:01:54 +0100] "GET /support/ HTTP/1.0" - -
  "http://www.s1.de/index.html" "Mozilla/4.6 [en] (Win98; I)"
Isis138.urz.uni-duesseldorf.de - - 01/Sep/1999:00:02:17 +0100] "GET /support/laserjet-support.html
  HTTP/1.0" - - "http://www.s4.de/support/" "Mozilla/4.0 (compatible; MSIE
  5.0; Windows 98; QXW0330d)"
hs2-210.handshake.de - - [01/Sep/1999:00:02:20 +0100] "GET /support/esc.html HTTP/1.0" - -
  "http://www.s1.de/support/" "Mozilla/4.6 [en] (Win98; I)"
pC19F2927.dip.t-dialin.net - - [01/Sep/1999:00:02:21 +0100] "GET /support/ HTTP/1.0" - -
  "http://www.s1.de/" "MOZILLA/4.5[de]C-CCK-MCD QXW03207 (WinNT;
  I)"
hs2-210.handshake.de - - [01/Sep/1999:00:02:22 +0100] "GET /service/notfound.html HTTP/1.0" -
  - "http://www.s1.de/support/esc.html" "Mozilla/4.6 [en] (Win98; I)"
hs2-210.handshake.de - - [01/Sep/1999:00:03:11 +0100] "GET /service/supportpack/ in
  dex_content.html HTTP/1.0" - - "http://www.s1.de/support/" "Mozilla/4.6
  [en] (Win98; I)"
hs2-210.handshake.de - - [01/Sep/1999:00:03:43 +0100] "GET /service/supportpack/kontakt.html
  HTTP/1.0" - - "http://www.s1.de/service/supportpack/index_content.html"
  "Mozilla/4.6 [en] (Win98; I)"
cache-dm03.proxy.aol.com - - [01/Sep/1999:00:03:57 +0100] "GET /support/ HTTP/1.0" - -
  "http://www.s1.de/" "Mozilla/4.0 (compatible; MSIE 5.0; AOL 4.0; Windows
  98; DigExt)"

Fig. 2. Excerpt from a Server Logfile

Table 1. URL Address and Code for the Address

URL Address	Code
www.s1.de/index.html	A
www.s1.de/support/	B
www.s1.de/support/esc.html	C
www.s1.de/support/service-not found.html	D
www.s1.de/service/supportpack/index_content.html	E
www.s1.de/service/supportpack/kontakt.html	F

Table 2. User, Time and Path the User has taken on the Web-Site

User Name	Time	Path
USER_1	1:54	A
USER_1	2:20 -2:22	B → C
USER_1	3:11	B
USER_1	3:43 - 3:44	E → F

3.2 User Entry Data / Profiles

On-line forms on a website are a very popular media for the acquisition of data from
visitors. Usually the website visitor is requested to fill in into these forms information
like name, address, telephone number etc. but also life style information and user

interests are stored. This information can be directly stored into a data base which can be taken later on for data mining. However, for a user it is often boring to answer all these questions. Therefore, on-line forms or questionnaires should be set up in such a way that they do not take too much of the user's time and that he is motivated to give all the requested answers.

A newer trend is the Open Profiling Standard (OPS) [3] which allows to automatically access user profiles from the browser of the client site. The OPS standard defines the data format and the transaction rules for electronic profiles [11]. The user can set up his profile on a voluntary basis and by doing so keep track of what information he likes to provide. The other advantage of an electronic profile for the user is that he only needs to define his basic profile once and not whenever he is entering a web site.

3.3 Web Documents and Web Meta Data

The web documents (HTML documuent, see Fig. 3) contain information such as text, images, video or audio. They have a structure that allows to recognize for e.g. the title of the page, the author, keywords and the main body. The formatting instruction must be removed in order to access the information that we want to mine on these sides. An example of an HTML document is given in Figure 3. The relevant information on this page is marked with grey color. Everything else is HTML code which is enclosed into brackets <>. The title of a page can be identified by searching the page for the code <title> to find the beginning of the title and for the code </title> to find the end of the title. Images can be identified by searching the webpage for the file extension .gif, .jpg.

Web meta data give us the topology of a website. This information is normally stored as a side-specific index table implemented as a directed graph. Usually, these web meta data are specified manually by the website administrator. This can become hard for large websites. Therefore, recently methods have been developed to annotate this documents automatically.

4 Data Mining

4.1 Basic Problem Types

Data Mining [4] methods can be distinguished into two main categories of data mining problems:

1. prediction and
2. knowledge discovery.

While prediction is the strongest goal, knowledge discovery is the weaker approach and usually prior to prediction.

The classification of a customer into a customer who is highly likely to buy a product belongs to predictive data mining. In this example, we have to mine a data base for a set of rules that describes the profile of a customer who has a preference for a certain product. The shop assistant can use this classification knowledge to identify a customer as a potential buyer.

```
<html>
<head>
        <title>welcome to the homepage of Petra Perner</title>
</head>

<body bgcolor="#ccffcc" text="black"
background="../images/hint.gif" link="#666699">

<td width="20" valign="top"><img height="5" width="20"
src="../images/nix.gif"></td>

<td width="423" valign="top">
<font face="Arial,Helvetica,Geneva" size="4" color="#666699">

Welcome to the homepage of Petra Perner</b><br></font></br></br>

<font face="Arial,Helvetica,Geneva" size="3"
color="#666699">Industrial Conference Data Mining 24.7.-25.7.2001
</font></br></br> </br>

<font face="Arial,Helvetica,Geneva" size="3" color="black">

In connection with MLDM2001 there will be held an industrial
conference on Data Mining.</br></br>
Please visit our website http://www.data-mining-forum.de for more
information.</br></br>
List of Accepted Papers for MLDM is now available. Information on
MLDM2001 you can find on this site under the link MLDM2001</br>
</br>

        </font></td></tr></table></div>
        </body>
</html>
```

Fig. 3. Example of an Html-Document

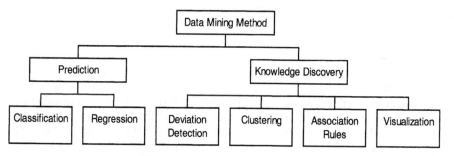

Fig. 4. Types of Data Mining Methods

For that kind of data mining, we need to know the classes or goals our system should predict. In most cases we might know these goals a-priori. However, there are other tasks were the goals are not known a-priori. In that case, we have to find out the classes based on methods such as clustering before we can go into predictive mining. Furthermore, the prediction methods can be distinguished into classification and regression while knowledge discovery can be distinguished into: deviation detection, clustering, mining association rules, and visualization. To categorize the actual problem into one of these problem types is the first necessary step when dealing with Data Mining.

Note that Figure 4 only describes the basic types of data mining methods. We consider for e.g. text mining, web mining or image mining only as variants of the basic types of data mining which need a special data preparation.

4.2 Prediction

4.2.1 Classification

Assume there is a set of observations from a particular domain. Among this set of data there is a subset of data labeled by class 1 and another subset of data labeled by class 2. Each data entry is described by some descriptive domain variables and the class label. To give the reader an idea, let us say we have collected information about customers, such as marital status, sex, and number of children. The class label is the information whether the customer has purchased a certain product or not. Now we want to know how the group of buyers and non-buyers is characterized.

The task is now to find a mapping function that allows to separate samples belonging to class 1 (e.g. the group of internet users) from those belonging to class 2 (e.g. the group of people that do not use the internet). Furthermore, this function should allow to predict the class membership of new formerly unseen samples.

Such kind of problems belong to the problem type "classification". There can be more than two classes but for simplicity we are only considering the two-class problem. The mapping function can be learnt by decision tree or rule induction, neural networks, discriminate analysis or case-based reasoning. We will concentrate in this paper on symbolic learning methods such as decision tree induction. The decision tree learnt based on the data of our little example described above is shown in Figure 5. The profile of the buyers is: marital_status = single, number_of_ children=0. The profile of the non-buyers is: marital_status = married or marital_status = single and number_of_children > 0. This information can be used to promote potential customers.

4.2.2 Regression

Whereas classification determines the set membership of the samples, the answer of regression is numerical. Suppose we have a CCD sensor. We give light of a certain luminous intensity to this sensor. Then this light is transformed into a gray value by the sensor according to a transformation function. If we change the luminous intensity we also change the gray value. That means the variability of the output variable, will be explained based on the variability of one or more input variables.

age	sex	marital_status	number of_children	purchaised
33	female	single	0	0
34	female	single	1	1
35	female	married	2	1
36	female	married	0	1
29	female	single	0	0
30	male	single	0	0
31	male	single	1	1
32	male	single	2	1
33	male	married	0	1

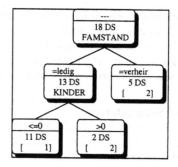

Fig. 5. Example Data Base and Resulting Decision Tree for Campaign Management

4.3 Knowledge Discovery

4.3.1 Deviation Detection
Real-world observation are random events. The determination of characteristic values such as the quality of an industrial part, the influence of a medical treatment to a patient group or the detection of visual attentive regions in images can be done based on statistical parameter tests.

4.3.2 Cluster Analysis
A number of objects that are represented by a n-dimensional attribute vector should be grouped into meaningful groups. Objects that get grouped into one group should be as similar as possible. Objects from different groups should be as dissimilar as possible. The basis for this operation is a concept of similarity that allows us to measure the closeness of two data entries and to express the degree of their closeness.

   Once groups have been found we can assign class labels to these groups and label each data entry in our data base according to its group membership with the corresponding class label. Then we have a data base which can serve as basis for classification.

4.3.3 Visualization
The famous remark "A picture is worth more than thousand words." especially holds for the exploration of large data sets. Numbers are not easy to overlook by humans. The summarization of these data into a proper graphical representation may give humans a better insight into the data. For example, clusters are usually numerically represented. The dendrogram illustrates these groupings, and gives a human an understanding of the relations between the various groups and subgroups.

   A large set of rules is easier to understand when structured in a hierarchical fashion and graphical viewed such as in form of a decision tree.

4.3.4 Association Rules
To find out associations between different types of information which seem to have no semantic dependence, can give useful insights in e.g. customer behavior.

Marketing manager have found that customers who buy oil in a supermarkt will also by vegetables. Such information can help to arrange a supermarket so that customers feel more attracted to shop there.

To discover which HTML documents are retrieved in connection with other HTML documents can give insight in the user profile of the website visitors.

4.3.5 Segmentation

Suppose we have mined a marketing data base for user profiles. In the next step we want to set up a mailing action in order to advertise a certain product for which it is highly likely that it attracts this user group. Therefore, we have to select all addresses in our data base that meet the desired user profile. By using the learnt rules as query to the data base we can segment our data base into customers that do not meet the user profile and into those that meet the user profile. The separation of the data into those data that meet a given profile from those that do not met a given profile is called segmentation. It can be used for a mailing action where only the address of the customers who meet a given profile are selected and mailed out an advertising letter.

5 Intelligent E-marketing with Data Mining and User-Adapted Interfaces

5.1 Objectives

In the following we describe the recent work we are developing for an on-line sales and advertisement model methods and processes for integrated Data Mining and the ensuing user-specific adaptation of the web contents. The result shall be tools comprising the following essential steps:

- Identification and recording of web data that are in the following steps the base for building up user profiles.
- Analysis of the data by data mining processes in order to discover and build up user profiles, e.g. correlation of activities like purchase of associated products or combining the purchase of some products with certain delivery options.
- Integration and visualization, respectively, of the analyzed data for the Web Content Management and the author process, respectively.
- Conversion of the user profiles and the set of rules into user-adapted multimedia presentations and interaction forms.

The solutions achieved in this project are to be new Data Mining processes, oriented on the Web-Mining, and allowing at the same time the feedback according to the knowledge drawn from the Data Mining process to the web contents and the Content Management, respectively. In the framework of this project we want to investigate among other things the connection of temporary user modeling with long-term models, as well as the reciprocal influence of both models in different application contexts and we want to realize them with the help of component technologies. As a result there will be prototypical software components at disposal.

5.2 The Architecture

Figure 6 describes the architecture of the E-shop system with integrated data mining components. These components include components to access data, clean data, data mining components, components to visualize the results of the data mining process and components for the direct usage of the mined knowledge in the e-shop.
In detail these functional components are:

- The user interface client components,
- The user modeling components
- The data mining components,
- The knowledge repository,
- The visualization component for the web usage mining and user profiles and
- The data base with the different media elements and templates.

The data are collected by on-line forms, by server logs and by cookie logs or java agents in a history list. This information is given as an input to the data mining component where it can be used for different purposes. The data can be used to learn the user model and the user preferences as well as the usage of the website. In the data mining component are realized data mining methods such as decision tree induction and conceptual clustering for attribute-value based and graph-structured data. Decision tree induction requires that the data have a class label. Conceptual clustering can be used to learn groups of similar data. When the groups have been discovered the data can be labeled by a group name and as such it can be used for decision tree induction to learn classification knowledge.

Based on the user model the presentation style and the content of the web site (adaptive multimedia product presentation) are controlled. Besides that the user model is used to set up specific marketing actions such as e.g. mailing actions or cross-selling actions. The results of the webusage mining are used to improve the website organization as well as for monitoring the impact rate of the advertisement of particular events. Product models and preferences are used to control the content of the website. The preferences can be learned based on the user´s navigation data. Besides that an intelligent dialogue component allows to control the dialogue with the user [9].

The following processes can be handled with these components:

- Web-Site Administration,
- Advertisement,
- Marketing and Selling,
- Adaptive Multimedia Product Presentation,
- Event Recognition, and
- Learning Ontology Knowledge.

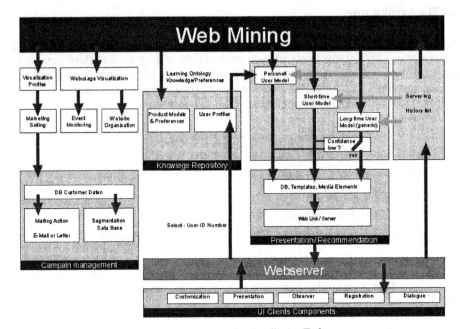

Fig. 6. Architecture of an intelligent E-shop

5.2.1 The Data

The data are the server log, the history list and the user data obtained by the registration component. The server log contains data described in Sect. 3.1. Data for the history list are collected by an observation component which is installed in the browser on the client site when the user is visiting the website. These observation components observe actions of the user on the internet pages [17].

5.2.2 User Models

Different user models are contained in our architecture: the individual user model, the short-term user model, and the long-term user model.

The individual user model can be obtained by setting up electronic user profiles. The users needs and preferences can be collected by a questionnaire [12][16] when the user is entering the website or by accessing electronic profiles which can be accessed from the browser of the client site [11]. Theses profiles can be stored in a knowledge repository as individual user profile and each time the user visits the web site and identifies himself it can be used to present the user the content depending from his preferences and the used hardware and software facilities.

To fill out forms or questionnaires requires considerable user effort and the cooperation of the user. Since not every user likes to give out information about himself therefore, it should be possible to categorize the users into several user groups. Each user group represents a significant and large enough group of users sharing several properties together. Based on these user groups should be controlled the functions of the e-shop. The identification of the user groups can be done based on the users navigation behavior. The user's action while browsing a web site should be observed and should be used to learn the user profiles.

The users interest may change over time. Therefore the user model should adapt to this concept drift. A recent trend separates the user model into a short-term and a long term user model [13][14]. The short-term user model is based on highly specific information, whereas the long-term user model is based on more general information. The short-term model is learned from the most recent observations only. It represents user models, which can adjust more rapidly to the user's changing interests. If the short-term model can not classify the actual user at all, it is passed on to the long-term model which represents stereotypical user groups [19]. The purpose of the long-term model is to model the user's general preferences for certain products that could not be classified by the short-term model.

5.2.3 Mining for the User Model

Webb et al. [18] summarize four major issue in learning user models:

- The need for large data sets;
- The need for labeled data;
- Concept drift, and
- Computational complexity.

The problem of the limited data set and the problem of concept drift has lead to hybrid user models separated into a short-term and a long-term user model.

Most applications use the nearest neighbor method to model the short-term user model. This method searches for similar cases in a data base and applies the action associated to the nearest case to the actual problem. A specific problem of this method is the selection of the right attributes that describe the user profile and/or the set up of the feature weights [13] as well as the complexity. Bayesian classifiers are used for the long-term model [13].

We intend to use incrementally decision tree induction to learn both user models; the short-term and the long-term user model. It allows us to use the same development strategy for learning the models in both cases. This can be an important system feature. To overcome the limited data set problem we use boosting for building the short-term model. Decision tree induction can be used to learn the classification model as well as to cluster data. In contrast to nearest neighbor methods, decision tree induction generalizes over the data. This will give us a good understanding of the user modeling process [5].

Decision tree induction allows one to learn a set of rules and basic features necessary for the user modeling. The induction process does not only act as a knowledge discovery process, it also works as a feature selector, discovering a subset of features from the whole set of features in the sample set that is the most relevant to the problem solution. A decision tree partitions the decision space recursively into sub-regions based on the sample set. In this way the decision tree recursively breaks down the complexity of the decision space. The outcome has a format, which naturally presents the cognitive strategy of the human decision-making process. This satisfies our need for visualization and reporting the results to the marketing people.

A decision tree consists of nodes and branches. Each node represents a single test or decision. In the case of a binary tree, the decision is either true or false. Geometrically, the test describes a partition orthogonal to one of the coordinates of the decision space. The starting node is usually referred to as the root node. Depending on whether the result of a test is true or false, the tree will branch right or left to another node. Finally, a terminal node is reached (sometimes referred to as a leaf), and a decision is made on the class assignment. Also non-binary decision trees are used. In these trees more than two branches may leave a node, but again only one branch may enter a node. For any tree all paths lead to a terminal node corresponding to a decision rule of the "IF-THEN" form that is a conjunction (AND) of various tests.

The main tasks during decision tree learning can be summarized as follows: attribute selection, attribute discretization, splitting, and pruning. We will develop special methods for attribute discretization [6] that allow to discretize numerical attributes into more than two intervals during decision tree learning and to agglomerated categorical attribute values into supergroups. This leads to more compact trees with better accuracy. Besides that we will develop special pruning methods. Both techniques are necessary for the special kind of data and will be set up for the special needs of learning the user model.

To understand the concept drift, we will develop a method to compare the outcome of the decision tree induction process and to derive conclusions from it. This will give us a special technique to control the user model.

5.2.4 Web Usage Mining

Analyzing the server logs and the history list can help to understand the user behavior and the web structure, thereby improving the design of the website. Applying data mining techniques on access logs unveils interesting access patterns that can be used to restructure sites in more efficient groupings, pinpoint effective advertising locations, and target specific users for specific selling ads.

Methods for web usage analysis based on sequence analysis are described in [20]. We intent to develop conceptual clustering technique to understand the user accessing pattern. Classical clustering methods only create clusters but do not explain why a cluster has been established. Conceptual clustering methods build clusters and explain why a set of objects confirms a cluster. Thus, conceptual clustering is a type of learning by observations and it is a way of summarizing data in an understandable manner [7]. In contrast to hierarchical clustering methods, conceptual clustering methods build the classification hierarchy not only based on merging two groups. The algorithmic properties are flexible enough in order to dynamically fit the hierarchy to the data. This allows incremental incorporation of new instances into the existing hierarchy and updating this hierarchy according to the new instance.

We propose an algorithm that incrementally learns the organizational structure [8]. This organization scheme is based on a hierarchy and can be up-dated incrementally as soon as new cases are available. The tentative underlying conceptual structure of the access pattern is visually presented to the user. We have developed two approaches for clustering access patterns. Both are based on approximate graph subsumption. The first approach is based on a divide-and-conquer strategy whereas the second is based on a split-and-merge strategy which better allows to fit the hierarchy to the actual structure of the application, but requires more complex operations. The first approach uses a fixed threshold for the similarity values. The second approach uses an evaluation function for the grouping of the cases.

5.2.5 Reporting Tools

Although the outcome of the data mining component is a set of rules or a description of the clusters which can be directly used to control the functional components of the website or directly incorporated into the user modeling component. We also prefer to report the results of the data mining process in a form a system administrator or marketing person can use for further review of the results. Therefore we will integrate visualization components into our system that allow to visualize the resulting decision tree, the hierarchical representation of the conceptual clusters, and the statistics for the event marketing.

5.2.6 Knowledge Repository

In the knowledge repository are stored individual user profiles and product models and preferences. The individual user profile is created by the user with the help of the registration component of the user interface. It can be updated by the user itself or electronically by the data mining component after having analyzed the user data when visiting the website.

6 Conclusions

We have introduced a new architecture extending an e-shop into an intelligent e-marketing and selling platform which can adapt to user needs and preferences. The data which can be accessed during a user session as well as the method for analysing these data play an important role for achieving this goal. Therefore, we have reviewed the basic data that can be created during a customer session. Based on the kind of data and the wanted output the data mining methods are selected. We have reviewed the basic data mining methods and given an overview on what kind of method is eligible for the considered result. We have identified two types of data mining methods useful for our first set up of the intelligent e-shop. These are classifications based on decision tree induction and conceptual clustering. With these methods we can solve such problems as learning the user model, web usage mining for web site organization, campaign management, and event monitoring. The data might be labeled or might not have a label. In the latter case clustering is to use to learn similar groups and label them. Recently, we have continued to develop and implement the methods for decision tree induction and conceptual clustering. Each method will be implemented as a component with standard input and output interfaces that allows to assemble the components as far as will be needed for the particular e-shop.

Acknowledgment. Part of this work has been funded by the German Ministry of Economy and Technology. The funding is greatly acknowledged.

References

1. M. Stolpmann, On-line Marketing Mix, Kunden finden, Kunden binden im E-Business, Galileo Press, Bonn 1999.
2. Cooley, R., Mobasher, B., and Srivastava, J., Data Preparation for Mining World Wide Web Browsing Patterns, Knowledge and Information Systems, 1(1), 1999.
3. M. Merz, E-Commerce und E-Business, dpunkt.verlag Heidelberg, 2002.
4. J. Han and M. Kamber, Data Mining, Concepts and Techniques, Academic Press, San Diego, 2001
5. P. Perner, Data Mining on Multimedia Data, Springer Verlag in preparation
6. P. Perner and S. Trautzsch, Multinterval Discretization for Decision Tree Learning, In: Advances in Pattern Recognition, A. Amin, D. Dori, P. Pudil, and H. Freeman (Eds.), LNCS 1451, Springer Verlag 1998, S. 475-482.
7. D.H. Fisher, "Knowledge Acquisition via Incremental Clustering," Machine Learning, 2: 139-172, 1987.
8. P. Perner and G. Fiss, Conceptual Clustering of Graph-structured Data, PKDD2002, submitted
9. P. Cunningham, R. Bergmann, S. Schmitt, R. Traphöhner, S. Breen, and , B. Smyth, WEBSELL: Intelligent Sales Assistent for the World Wide Web, Zeitschrift Künstliche Intelligenz, 1, 2001, p. 28-32.
10. T. Ardissono and A. Goy, Tailoring the Interaction with Users in Web Stores, Journal on User Modeling and User-Adapted Interaction, 10(4) , 2000, p.251-303.
11. S. Shearin and P. Maes, Representation and Ownership of Electronic Profiles, Workshop Proc. Interactive Systems for 1-to-1 E-Commerce, CHI 2000, The Hague (The Netherlands), April 1-6, 2000.
12. S. Shearin and H. Liebermann, Intelligent Profiling by Example, Proc. of Intern. Conf. of Intelligent User Interfaces (IUI2001), p. 145-152, Santa Fe, NM, Jan. 14-17, 2001.
13. D. Billsus and M. Pazzani, A Hybrid User Model for News Story Classification, In: J. Kay, User Modeling: Proceedings of the Seventh International Conference, UM99, Springer Wien New York, 1999, p. 99-108.
14. J. Kay and R. Thomas, Long term learning in the workplace, Communications of the ACM, 38(7), July 1995, 61-69.
15. I. Koychev and I. Schwab, Adaption to Drifting User`s Interests,
16. Henry Lieberman. *Autonomous Interface Agents.* In Proceedings of ACM Conference on Human Factors in Computing Systems (CHI), 1997
17. M. Claypool, Phong Le, M. Waseda, D. Brown, Implicit Interest Indicators, IEEE Internet Computing, Nov./Dez. 2001 http://www.computer.org/internet
18. G.I. Webb, M.J. Pazzani, and D. Billsus, Machine Learning for User Modeling, User Modeling and User-Adapted Interaction, 11: 19-29, 2001.
19. J Kay, Lies, damned lies and stereotypes: pragmatic approximations of users, in Procs of UM94 - 1994 User Modeling Conference, UM Inc, Boston, USA, 1994, pp 175-184.
20. B. Masand and M. Spiliopoulou (Eds.) Web Usage Analysis and User Profiling, LNAI 1836, Springer Verlag 1999.

The indiGo Project: Enhancement of Experience Management and Process Learning with Moderated Discourses

Klaus-Dieter Althoff[1], Ulrike Becker-Kornstaedt[1], Björn Decker[1],
Andreas Klotz[2], Edda Leopold[2], Jörg Rech[1], and Angi Voss[2]

[1] Fraunhofer–Institut für Experimentelles Software Engineering (IESE), Sauerwiesen 6,
67661 Kaiserslautern
{althoff, becker, decker, rech}@iese.fraunhofer.de
[2] Fraunhofer–Institut für Autonome Intelligente Systeme (AIS), Schloss Birlinghoven,
53754 Sankt Augustin
{klotz, leopold, voss}@ais.fraunhofer.de

Abstract. Within this paper we describe the indiGo approach to preparation, moderation, and analysis of discourses to enhance experience management. In the indiGo project this has been exemplified for the process learning domain. indiGo includes an integration of approaches for e-participation, experience management, process modeling and publishing, as well as text mining. We describe both the methodology underlying indiGo and the indiGo platform. In addition, we compare indiGo to related work. Currently a case study is ongoing for an in-depth evaluation of the indiGo approach.

1 Introduction

Business process models of organizations operating in the innovative software industry are one of their major knowledge assets. However, these models need to be (a) constantly evaluated and revised in the business of those organizations as well as (b) enhanced by further knowledge to increase their applicability.

The approach of the BMBF funded project indiGo[1] is to support this evaluation and enhancement. It offers members of an organization (a) to engage in discourses about the process models itself or their execution and (b) presents process-related lessons learned, fitting to the current project context. On the organizational level, completed discourses are analyzed and summarized to improve related process models and capture lessons learned. To achieve these objectives, indiGo offers an integrated, comprehensive set of methods and a technical infrastructure as a joint effort of two Fraunhofer institutes: Fraunhofer IESE (Institute for Experimental Software

---

[1] indiGo (Integrative Software Engineering using Discourse-Supporting Groupware) is funded by the German "Ministerium für Bildung und Forschung" (BMBF) under grant number 01 AK 915 A (see http://indigo.fraunhofer.de)

P. Perner (Ed.): Advances in Data Mining 2002, LNAI 2394, pp. 53–79, 2002.

Engineering) in Kaiserslautern and Fraunhofer AIS (Autonomous Intelligent Systems) in Sankt Augustin.

The indiGo methods and tools add value through the speed-up of innovation cycles by involving a greater number of people and recording more information on processes in the form of discourses. In addition, they improve the construction of organizational knowledge through the preparation, moderation, and analysis of discourses supported by text mining and case-based reasoning. Current approaches to experience management are reinforced by providing a solution to integrate results of discourses into the experience base, a repository for business experiences.

The final indiGo technical infrastructure will consist of the Zeno® groupware tool of AIS, IESE's experience management environment INTERESTS, IESE's tool for process modeling and publishing Spearmint, as well as tools for text mining of discourses from AIS.

Both the developed methods and the indiGo architecture will be evaluated mid 2002 within a case study on process learning carried out at IESE. First results will be available in fall 2002.

In Chapters 3 and 4 we introduce the indiGo methodology and platform, respectively. Chapter 3 also includes a detailed process-learning example to exemplify the indiGo approach. Chapter 4 is also concerned with putting indiGo into context. For this, a terminological framework is presented in Chapter 2 and, based on this, the relevant state of the art is described. We then classify indiGo according to the framework. Finally, we give a short outlook on planned activities.

2   indiGo – The Framework

indiGo's key objective is to create and sustain living process models, that is, process models that are accepted by the organizations members, adapted to organizational changes on demand, and continuously enriched with experience from the operating business of the organization. Process learning requires at least four different kinds of knowledge in an organization: Process models (with their associated templates), experiences from instantiating process models in concrete projects, discussions about processes in closed or open groups, and private annotations of process models.

For example, assume Ms. Legrelle, a team leader in the organization, has to compose an offer for a subcontract from a small start-up. The process model for the acquisition of industrial projects has a subprocess devoted to the contract. It suggests that the payment scheme should not be too fine-grained in order to minimize administrative overhead. Ms. Legrelle feels uncomfortable with this guideline. The year before she had had a subcontract with another start-up, Hydra, which got bankrupt, so that the last payment was lost for her team although they had completed the work. Ms. Legrelle prefers to design the new offer with a frequent payment schedule, at the cost of more overhead in the administrative unit.

Clearly, Ms. Legrelle would not like to modify the organization's process model (1) for industrial project acquisition on her own - it is not her job and her view may be too subjective. She would probably agree that her experience with the Hydra project be recorded as a lesson to be learned, but even so, she would hardly take the trouble to fill in the required form to create an "official" case (2). Rather, she would like to suggest her exception from the guideline to her colleagues, backed up by the example of Hydra, and wait for their responses (3). Whatever the conclusion, she would probably add it as a personal note (4) to the guideline in the respective subprocess.

2.1 Knowledge Compaction, Usage, and Construction

indiGo takes into account all four categories of knowledge occurring in the previous example and supports them as successive stages in a process of knowledge compaction (aggregation, condensation, summarization, or classification). Figure 1 arranges the four knowledge categories on one layer and embeds it into layers of knowledge usage and knowledge construction.

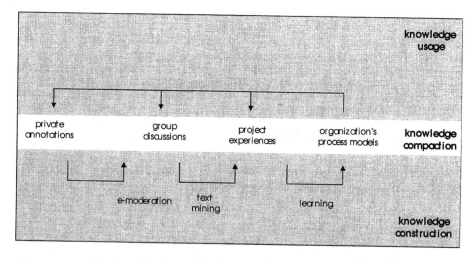

Fig. 1. Layers of knowledge compaction, usage and creation for process-centered applications

Knowledge compaction is the process of (a) decontextualization and (b) formalization with the goal of (c) decreasing modification times as well as increasing (d) lifetime, (e) obligingness, and (f) visibility. As indicators of knowledge compaction (a-f) are correlated, and they exhibit a clear progression from private annotations over group discussions, to lessons learned, and the organization's process models. Private annotations are highly contextualized, informal, secret, and non-binding, they have a short lifetime and can be updated often, while process models are highly decontextualized, formal, public, and obliging, they have a long lifetime and are updated infrequently.

One central issue in experience management is how to offer the right knowledge at the right time. As the domain of indiGo is based on process models, they should form the backbone for knowledge delivery. While applying (instantiating) a particular process model, members of the organization should find - a mouse click away - supplementary knowledge that is dynamically retrieved with regard to the users' current project context. This supplementary knowledge is provided through associated discussions in the users' groups and their private annotations and, of course, captures lessons learned from completed or current projects.

If no relevant knowledge is available, the user has encountered a gap in the knowledge and may write a quick private note that he can attach to the current part of the process model. In case he is a member of a group that is allowed to discuss this model he may raise the problem in the related discussion. Other users may be able to help, possibly they had been confronted with a similar problem formerly and had written a private note to remember the solution. Then they may bring this note into the group discussion.

Either-way, if a new solution or conclusion turns up and finds approval, it may be added as a new experience to the experience base. The process model would be adapted periodically as substantial feedback is accumulated from the discussions and the new experiences.

indiGo is more comprehensive than other approaches to organizational learning (Tautz 2000, Bergmann 2001, Kluge 1999, Minor & Staab 2002) because it bridges the gap between informal, communication-oriented knowledge and formal, organization-oriented knowledge and provides a socio-technical solution that covers individual knowledge usage as well as social knowledge creation.

3   indiGo – The Methodology

How an organization can accomplish process learning using the indiGo platform (its technical side) is the core of the indiGo methodology.

3.1   Introduction by Bootstrapping

The indiGo methodology is in itself structured in terms of a process model, called the indiGo model for process learning. The self description of the indiGo methodology through indiGo process models offers the opportunity to 'bootstrap' indiGo, that is, to apply indiGo to itself. First, it allows to have a test run of both the methodology and the technical infrastructure during the introduction of indiGo. Furthermore, since the persons involved in the indiGo introduction directly perform and experience this approach, it will be their prime interest to resolve occurring difficulties. Therefore, the members of the organization can rely on a tested infrastructure and a consolidated team to support them in the roll-out phase.

The bootstrap approach to introducing indiGo also implements three feedback cycles: A process-related, an organization-specific-methodic, and a general-methodic one. The process-related feedback cycle is the application of the indiGo methodology to the processes of the organization. The organization-specific-methodic one is the continuous improvement of the indiGo methodology at a specific organization. The general-methodic one is the feedback of experience gained by introducing the indiGo methodology by the supporting organizations, thus improving the generic process model of indiGo.

3.2 Process Learning Processes

The basic objective of the indiGo methodology is to create and sustain a living process model, that is, a process model that is (a) accepted by the organizations members, (b) adapted to organizational changes on demand, and (c) continuously enriched with experience from the operating business of the organization.

The processes of the indiGo model are ordered into three groups: Core processes, strategy processes, and support processes. Core processes generate a direct benefit for the organization: Creation of a process model, introduction of a process model, supporting process execution, and maintenance of a process model. Strategy processes cover the orientation and justification of the experience factory (EF) (Basili, Caldiera & Rombach 1994). This includes the definition or update of subject areas, setting objectives for the subject areas, and creating a short and long term perspective for the EF. Support processes assist core processes or strategy processes and include moderating discussions, processing lessons learned based on contributions to the discussion, handling feedback, managing the EF, and defining requirements for improving the technical infrastructure.

Besides this structure according to content of the processes, the process learning methodology differentiates two phases of process learning: First, in the *introduction phase*, the process model is first discussed on a hypothetical basis by the members of an organization. This phase focuses (a) on resolving potential conflicts associated with the new process description and (b) to elicit process improvement opportunities. At the end of the discussion, the results are summarized to improve the process model. If needed, this phase is augmented with a pilot application of the improved process model.

In the *operational phase*, the focus of the process learning processes is on detecting and solving problems revealed during process execution, that is, detecting and handling knowledge deficiencies. The (instantiated) methodology assures that certain members of the organization are responsible for this solution and that these solutions are preserved within the organization.

An instantiation of the indiGo methodology will be performed as follows: First, subject areas are defined and prioritized. The prioritization is used to select subject areas for the test run, the roll-out phase and future opportunities to enlarge the scope of process learning. Second, organization members are assigned to the roles and subject areas. Third, the generic process model of indiGo is instantiated to the needs of the organization by discussing them via the indiGo technical infrastructure. This discussions are continued throughout the application of the indiGo methodology, thus adapting and improving the processes of the indiGo methodology.

3.3 Role Model

The indiGo role model and subject areas together build a fine-grained framework that allows to adapt the indiGo methodology to the needs and settings of the organization. For each role involved, it describes a set of responsibilities that are performed by the respective role. This role model is complemented by a defined set of subject areas describing relevant areas of knowledge of the organization. Since the subject areas are organization-specific, they will not be detailed further. However, for the role model a description can be given at a generic level.

- The task of the *Members of the Organization* is to discuss the process models, report problems in process execution, and provide experience relevant for the processes. These contributions are further processed by the members of the EF team.
- The *Moderator* facilitates the discussion of the members of the organization. S/he holds close contact to the Process Owner and Authors to start discussions with relevant topics. From time to time, the moderator summarizes the discussion to help new organizational members to catch-up with the discussion. In the end of a discussion, the moderator also creates a summary for the EF team and the process owner.
- The *Process Owner* is responsible for a set of processes, often about a certain subject area. Due to his/her position within the organization, the Process Owner is allowed to take decisions about the definition and content of a process. Examples for such positions are the upper management for core processes of an organization or the provider of a certain service for support processes.
- The *Process Author* is responsible for creating and maintaining process descriptions as a whole or parts of it. If not performed by the same person, the Process Author supports the Process Owner by preparing decisions of the process owner.

These roles are supported by the EF team, which is presented in the following list (Feldmann, Frey et al. 2000). It is possible to assign several roles in the EF team to one person, thus lowering the dedicated resources.

- The Process Engineer is the expert for process-related issues. In the context of the indiGo methodology, the Process Engineer captures process information from process experts as well as from available process documents and process artifacts, and structures this information into a process model. The Process Engineer must have knowledge on process improvement methods, such as process assessments. Furthermore, a Process Engineer must have familiarity with existing process standards.
- The *Experience Manager* is responsible for maintaining and improving the quality of experience in the reuse repository. S/he assesses the existing measurement of experience quality and sets new measurement goals. Furthermore, the Experience Manager defines the reuse policy, that is, what kind of experience (gained during project execution) is to be reused.
- The *Experience Engineer* is responsible for extracting reusable experience gained during project execution. In addition, it is his/her responsibility to provide the development organization with reusable experience. S/he also assists in setting goals for projects, project planning, and experience packaging.
- The *Project Supporter* performs several tasks to support project execution. On the one hand, s/he serves as a consultant for the development organization by providing lessons learned and other forms of key corporate knowledge that are stored in the Experience Base. On the other hand, s/he is directly involved in project execution: Developing and maintaining measurement plans and supervising the data collection for the project. Furthermore, s/he s responsible for initiating,

planning, and controlling changes in the applied processes for process improvements or solving problems that have surfaced.

- The *Librarian* runs the Experience Base. S/he is responsible for entering data into the repository, and usually reports to the Experience Manager.

Furthermore, responsibilities for process learning activities are assigned to organization members outside the EF team that create synergies for those organizational members. This also lowers the need for dedicated resources and creates acceptance for the process learning activities.

3.4   Experimental Evaluation of indiGo

The methodology and tools developed for indiGo will be evaluated through a case study, which will be performed at Fraunhofer IESE starting in April 2002. First results should be available at the end of 2002. The organizational framework of the evaluation of the indiGo approach is as follows.

IESE's approximately 100 regular staff do applied research, evaluation and transfer of software engineering methods and techniques in a broad range of industrial and publicly funded projects. IESE's knowledge management is performed by the CoIN-Team (CoIN = Corporate Information Network) with five part-time members. They maintain a process model database (CoIN-IQ) and a database of lessons learned from current and completed projects (CoIN-EF). The process models are partitioned into subject areas, for instance project-related matters are distinguished from cooperation with universities, and persons concerned with the subjects in the organization are selected as owners of the respective process models. Lessons learned from the projects are elicited by the CoIN-team, which also provides the Process Engineer.

The process models concerned with project management need to be adapted to a recent restructuring of IESE. As projects are the core business of IESE, the new process models are central for the organization and affect most of the staff. It is vital that they accept and "live" the new process models and cooperate to continuously improving them. Due to the variety of the projects, the processes can reasonably be captured at an abstract level only. That means, the instantiation of the abstract process models is highly knowledge-intensive.

In a series of workshops, which involved the higher management, an initial revision of the process descriptions was elaborated. Through regular informal contacts it was assured that the higher management would support the introduction of the new processes. Process models with a high potential of conflicts will be introduced in April 2002 according to the indiGo methodology.

The process of creating project offers is planned to be introduced in two phases: A discussion phase and a pilot phase. In the discussion phase members of the organization discuss the process description without actually instantiating it. This will elicit not only suggestions on the process descriptions, but related stories or examples from their daily work. A member of the CoIN-team or an independent moderator will facilitate the discussion. The author of the process description will point out topics to lead the discussion in a goal-oriented way. The participants are asked to indicate the type of their contributions by using a set of labels that were specially designed for the case study. The use of labels stimulates a rational and easier to understand argumentation. In case of need the moderator will contact experts to comment on a contribution. For example, the lawyer could answer questions on the new laws of warranty that became effective at the beginning of this year. On terminating the discussion phase, the process author and the responsible person from the CoIN-team will secure the contributions. Extracted experiences have to be approved by the responsible process owner before they are transferred to the experience base. In some cases, further focused investigations, like a project analysis, will be taken into consideration (Tautz 2000). Text mining methods for clustering contributions or adding semantic links will enhance the analysis conducted by both, the process author and the experience engineer. Selected contributions, especially open arguments, will remain with the process model.

In the subsequent pilot phase the process descriptions will be evaluated at daily work. Now practical problems will turn up that have to be solved by the staff or some experts. These discussions, too, will be evaluated for improving the process descriptions and extending the experience base. Clearly, the emphasis will now lie on gathering experiences while the process model will stabilize.

Finally, the revised process description will be published for regular operation. Due to the comprehensive validation during the discussion and pilot phases the number of new contributions is expected to be small. Therefore, the responsible process author may monitor the discussion with low effort beside their other tasks. For the process of writing project offers, this would be the administrative person whose work will be alleviated through efficient instantiations of the process model. Supported by text mining services the responsible moderator will continue to observe the discussions in order to identify interesting experiences and projects that require further analysis. If problems of executing the process models are starting to accumulate a new revision will be scheduled.

4   indiGo – The Software Platform

The indiGo technical platform integrates two independent types of systems for a completely new service. While one system acts as a source for documents, like descriptions of business process models, the other acts as a source for related information, like private annotations, public comments or lessons and examples from an experience base. Currently the business process model repository CoIN-IQ acts as the document source, related information is provided either by the groupware Zeno or the lessons learned repository CoIN-EF.

As shown in Figure 2 the indiGo platform, as presented at CeBIT 2002, consists of three core components. The integrator acts as a middleware between the document and information source. On the left hand side CoIN-IQ hosts the business process models that can be supported by information from the second system. Zeno on the right side manages annotations and discussions about the business process models from CoIN-IQ.

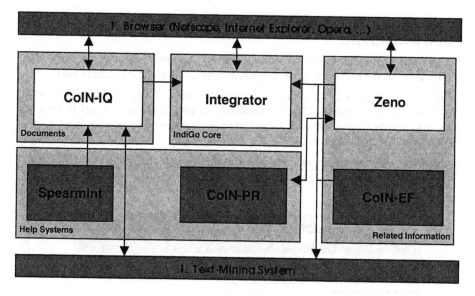

Fig. 2. Information flow in the indiGo platform (upper level presented at CeBIT 2002)

To enhance the functionality of indiGo we connected Zeno with CoIN-PR (CoIN Project Registry), a project information repository that stores all data about the projects and associated users. Information about the projects include, for example, the project type (e.g., research & development, transfer or consulting), status, funding, project staff, project manager or the list of participating partners. CoIN-PR delivers information about a specific user's current projects, which is used to index contributions in Zeno with a project context and to construct queries for CoIN-EF. Besides commenting the business process models, the user has the opportunity to recall context-specific lessons learned from CoIN-EF.

To support and enhance the various roles in indiGo text-mining tools will be applied to analyze the discussions in order to detect new, previously unknown or hidden information for moderators and other roles, especially with the goal to extend or improve the lessons learned and the process models.

Based on standard internet technology indiGo is a truly distributed system. While Zeno is hosted on a web server at Fraunhofer AIS in Sankt Augustin, Germany, the CoIN system family is located at and maintained by Fraunhofer IESE in Kaiserslautern, Germany.

4.1   The indiGo Integrator

The integrator is the glue between a document server like CoIN-IQ and a server for related information like Zeno. It provides an integrated view upon a document and related information. Based on Perl the integrator is a CGI script that offers three fundamental functions that are called either by CoIN-IQ or Zeno:

- Discuss: This function creates a split view upon a document and related information. In the current indiGo context this is a view on the specific business process model from CoIN-IQ in the upper part and beneath the appropriate discussion from Zeno.

- Annotate: Analogous to the previous function, the integrator creates a split view upon a business process model and a personal annotation for the current user.

- Destroy: To work with only one system this function collapses the split view of indiGo to a single frame. This is particularly helpful if the user wants to turn off the discussions from Zeno or if he switches into another discourse in Zeno that is not related to business processes.

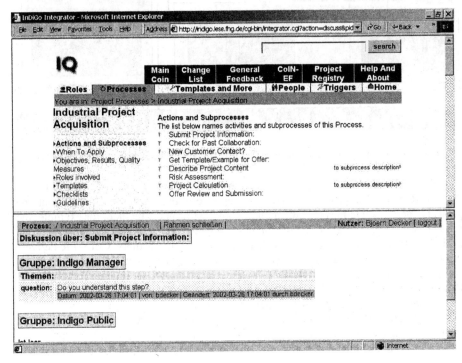

Fig. 3. Split View with CoIN-IQ at the top and a Related Discussion in Zeno beneath

4.2 CoIN-IQ

CoIN-IQ is IESE's business process model repository. The topics currently covered range from core processes (e.g., project set-up and execution) to support processes (e.g., using the IESE information research service) to research focused processes (e.g., performing Ph.D. work at IESE). Based on the results of a diploma thesis performed in advance, the build-up of CoIN-IQ in 2000 took about ten person months of effort. This effort was equally distributed between the technical realization and the creation of content for CoIN-IQ. About four person months of effort are allocated in 2001 for further content build-up and maintenance.

For the whole CoIN, CoIN-IQ has particular function for the integration of services within IESE's knowledge management activities: (a) They are used to define the point in the business processes execution where services (like knowledge acquisition or access to sources) are performed. (b) They describe the usage of services and knowledge management activities themselves (e.g., like project touch down analyses).

The content and infrastructure is created and maintained by the CoIN team, a team of scientists working for CoIN on a part-time basis. The CoIN team either performs those activities themselves, or distributes them among other IESE members. The latter will gain even more importance when the indiGo system is running, since the CoIN team will ensure that the result of the discussions are (a) used to improve the process model or (b) analyzed and appropriate lessons learned distilled from them.

4.2.1   Objectives of CoIN-IQ

The objectives of CoIN-IQ can be positioned according to four criteria: (1) The purpose of process models, (2) the origin and (3) usage of the process models, and (4) the modeling techniques. In summary, CoIN-IQ uses structured text describing empirical and theoretical process models to be executed by human agents. This is detailed in the following.

For the general purpose of process models, Curtis, Kellner, and Over (1992) identify five different categories: Facilitate human understanding and communication, support process improvement, support process management, automate process guidance, and automate execution. According to this classification scheme, CoIN-IQ fits into the first category of facilitating human understanding and communication: The processes are executed by human agents (i.e., IESE members), based on the process description. Supporting and enforcing process execution beyond this human-based approach (e.g., by workflow modeling and enactment as in Maurer and Holz (1999)) was regarded as non-suitable for the purposes of IESE due to the creative nature of its business processes. Furthermore, processes according to the process models are executed rather infrequently (< 10 times per month), therefore (a) automation of the processes was not supposed to leverage a high cost/benefit and (b) tracking of process status can be done by asking the responsible process executor. In addition, the experience made with the Electronic Process Guide (EPG) (Becker-Kornstaedt & Verlage 1999) showed that web-based process descriptions are a feasible way of distributing process knowledge within creative environments such as software business. In particular, changes to web-based process models can be communicated much quicker than paper-based process models, thus enabling quick integration of experience.

The origin of process models can be empirical (i.e., based on actual processes (Bandinelli, Fugetta et. al 1995)) and theoretical (i.e., reflecting a planned process execution). Process models in CoIN-IQ have both origins: Some of the process models reflect well-established processes (like, e.g., the administrative project set-up), others represent new procedures (e.g., the reflection of recent changes in the organizational structure of IESE).

The usage of process models can be descriptive (i.e., a description of a process) or prescriptive (i.e., intended to be used as an instruction for process execution). The process models within CoIN-IQ are prescriptive with different degrees of obligation. In general, administrative procedures (e.g., project accounting) have to be followed without exception; best-practice process models like project management procedures are to be seen as recommendations.

The process modeling technique of CoIN-IQ is structured text, which is due to several reasons: Zero effort training, straightforward modeling, and perpetuation in industrial strength applications. Zero effort has to be spent on training, since any IESE member can read structured text without previous training. Furthermore, straightforward modeling means that any IESE members can model processes using structured text, if supported by guidelines and the CoIN team. This aspect is additionally fortified by the experience in scientific publishing of most IESE members.

4.2.2   Content of CoIN-IQ

To achieve these objectives, the following information is captured within CoIN-IQ. Each of those information objects can be linked to other objects according to Figure 4:

- *Process Descriptions*: Process descriptions describe the activities captured within CoIN (e.g., project management). Complex processes are structured into a hierarchy of super- and sub-processes.
- *Role Descriptions*: Role descriptions describe the roles that are involved in the execution of processes.
- *Agent Descriptions*: Agent Descriptions are used within role descriptions to name roles that are performed by a specific IESE member.
- *Product Representations*: A Product Representation represents a document to be used during process execution.

  Overviews: Overviews structure the other objects within CoIN-IQ to facilitate browsing.

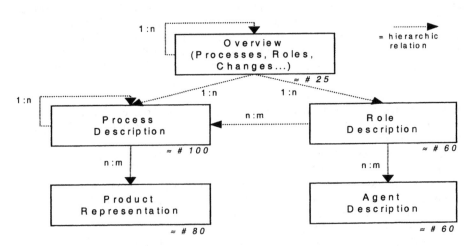

Fig. 4. Simplified structure of objects in CoIN-IQ. Arrows show how objects are linked. The relations are to be read according to the direction of the arrows (e.g., one overview can refer to n other overviews, role descriptions or process descriptions). Italics denominate the number of elements of the respective type of objects within CoIN-IQ.

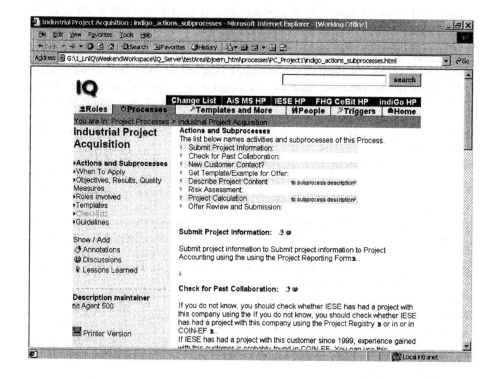

Fig. 5. Screenshot of a process description. (Figure shows anonymized demonstrator)

The discussion in indigo are related to Process Descriptions in CoIN-IQ. Therefore, they are described in the following. As depicted in Figure 5, a process within CoIN-IQ is described according to the following structure: "Actions and Subprocesses", "When to apply?", "Objectives, Results, and Quality Measures", "Roles involved", "Templates", "Checklists", and "Guidelines". The content and purpose of these sections are described in the following:

- *"Actions and Subprocesses"* describe the steps of the process execution. In CoIN-IQ, a distinction is made between actions and sub-processes. Actions are atomic steps that are not refined any further. Sub-processes are described in a separate process description according to this structure. The super-process contains a link to the sub-process, followed by a short explanation of the sub-process content.

- *"When to Apply"* gives a short overview of a process' context, thus helping the user to determine if the current process description is the desired one. To facilitate this overview even more, it is again structured into three sub-sections: Scope, Trigger and Viewpoint. "Scope" contains one or two sentences about the thematic range of a process and thus, the content of a process description. "Trigger" as the second sub-section describes the condition that starts the execution of a process. These triggering conditions can be events released from outside IESE (e.g., a customer telephone call), dependencies with other process executions (e.g., start or finish of a process) or dependencies from product states (e.g., a deliverable is about to be finished). "Viewpoint" contains the role from whose view the process is described.

- *"Objectives, Results and Quality Measures"* is information intended to guide the execution of a process. The difference between the three sub-sections is the increasing degree of quantification of quality information. "Objectives" are general objectives of the process. "Results" are tangible outcomes of the process (e.g., meeting minutes). "Quality Measures" describe properties of such results (e.g., the number of pages of the meeting minutes should range between 10 and 20) or the process itself (e.g., the effort spent on preparing a meeting should not exceed one person day).
- *"Roles involved"* provides an overview of the roles involved in the process and links the Role Descriptions. An experienced user can find quickly the Role Descriptions that are distributed within the "Actions and Subprocesses" and "Guidelines" Section.
- *"Templates"* lists the products referenced by the process description. This overview is intended to support IESE members who are accustomed to the process and just need quick access to artifacts.
- *"Checklists"* is also intended for the experienced user. It summarizes important steps and results of the Process Description.
- *"Guidelines"* give hints for performing a process, like "do's and don'ts" or frequently asked questions about a process. Furthermore, frequently used variances of a process are modeled as guidelines. This reduces the number of similar process descriptions and lowers the effort to maintain the process description. Each guideline has a "speaking headline" in the form of a question or statement, followed by explanatory text.

4.2.3   CoIN-IQ for indiGo

To be part of the indiGo platform, CoIN-IQ was subject to substantial changes. First, the web-pages of CoIN-IQ were re-designed due to usability criteria. Second, buttons for private annotations, group discussions and lessons learned related to a specific process or process element were inserted into these web-pages. Third, the homepage of CoIN-IQ was copied into ZENO, this allowing to show user-specific announcements on these pages like new articles since the last login.

4.2.4   Process Model Editors and Publishing Software

Spearmint is IESE's process modeling environment (Becker-Kornstaedt, Hamann et al. 1999). A Spearmint process model can be published on the web as an electronic process guide (EPG) with the process guidance tool EPG (Kellner, Becker-Kornstaedt et al. 1998). In the course of this transformation relationships such as product flow, role assignment, or refinement are converted into hyperlinks, and the information described in the attributes appears as text in the EPG. To customize EPGs, the attributes to be generated can be specified. If a process model has been modified, the EPG can be regenerated easily. CoIN-IQ is an instance of such an EPG.

In the following, based on Dellen, Könnecker, and Scott (2000), relevant process modeling editors and publication software are summarized. From the perspective of process learning, three kinds of tools can be distinguished:

(a) Software that publishes the process model in a representation that is understandable to humans,

(b) software that additionally allows to annotate or discuss process models, and

(c) software that focuses on the collaborative creation of process models, that is, process engineers and authors can create and manipulate process models.

While (a) is a passive way of communicating process models that have to be complemented by organizational measures to induce real change, (b) allows a two-way communication between process engineer or author and organizational members. (c) concentrates on supporting process engineers and authors in the creation of process models, which in practice will also include discussions.

For each of those categories, Table 1 gives some examples. Process Model (No 1) belongs to category (a). It is focused in business process design and improvement of ISO 9000 processes. For category (b), a prototype extension of Spearmint was developed to gain some first experiences with annotations and discussion on a private, groupwise, and public level (No 3). Furthermore, PageSeeder can be used to augment the HTML representation generated from the process modes (EPG) (Scott, Jeffery & Becker-Kornstaedt 2001) (No 4). DaimlerChrysler's LID-system (von Hunnius 2000) allows public annotation of software process models, which the process engineer can distill to lessons learned and attached to the process model (No 5). Finally, as representatives of category (c) ADONIS (No 6) and ARIS Web Designer (No 10) focus on collaborative editing and publishing of graphical represented business process models. ARIS also offers support for enacting the business process models, for instance, via Lotus Notes.

Table 1. Overview of process modeling and publication software

Name	No	Publica tion	Annot ation	Discus sion	Coll. Creation	URL / further information
Process Model	1	X				www.processmodel.com
Process	2	X				www.scitor.com/pv3/purchase.proces.asp
SPEARMINT / Annotation	3	X	X	X		www.iese.fhg.de/Spearmint_EPG/
SPEARMINT / PageSeeder	4	X	X	X		www.iese.fhg.de/Spearmint_EPG/
LID System	5	X	X	X		(von Hunnius (2000))
ADONIS	6	X			X	www.boc-eu.com
INCOME	7	X			X	www.promatis.de
INNOVATOR	8	X			X	www.mid.de
in-Step	9	X			X	www.microtool.de
Aris Web Designer	10	X			X	www.ids-scheer.de
Aris Web Publisher	11	X				www.ids-scheer.de

4.3   Zeno

Turning from tools for process models to tools for discussion, the objectives and major concepts of Zeno can be motivated.

4.3.1   Software for Document-Centered Discourses on the Web

Zeno is an e-participation platform (www.e-partizipation.org) (Voss 2002) with a spectrum of functions that comprises and extends
(a) simple threaded discussions
(b) document-centered discourses
(c) information structuring during group decision making

Most electronic discussion forums, like the ones mentioned above but also newsgroups, support simple threaded discussions (a). Some tools, e.g. http://icommons.harvard.edu/, recognize URLs or even HTML tags in the contributions or allow to attach documents.

D³E belongs to category (b). It can process any hierarchical HTML file into a frames-based environment with automatic hyperlinking for navigating around sections, checking citations and footnotes, and tight integration with a discussion space for critiquing documents. Moderators may influence the look and feel of a discussion space, they may edit, hide, or delete contributions. D3E is available as open source (http://d3e.sourceforge.net/) (Sumner & Buckingham Shum 1998). The e-learning platforms Hyperwave eLearning SUITE supports annotations and discussions of course units. Moreover, it offers a set of labels to characterize contributions as notes, questions, responses, acceptance and rejection (www.hyperwave.com).

Predefined labels for qualifying contributions are more familiar in tools for group decision making (c), especially for brainstorming (www.facilitate.com). Softbicycle's QuestMap (www.softbicycle.com) distinguishes questions, ideas, pros, cons, decisions, notes, and references, a variant of the famous IBIS grammar (Kunz & Rittel 1970) which was first implemented in gIBIS (Conklin & Begemann 1988). Tools in this category usually allow to restructure the contributions, i.e. they support maps rather than threads, deliberative argumentation rather than spontaneous reaction.

The first version of Zeno, which also supported a variant of IBIS (Gordon & Karakapilidis 1999), was presented at CeBIT 1996 and continuously improved up to version 1.9 in 1999. Since then a completely new system has been realized addresses a broader spectrum of discourses in the knowledge society: Participatory problem solving, consensus building (Voss, Röder & Wacker 2002), mediated conflict resolution (Märker, O., Hagedorn, H., Trénel, M. & Gordon 2002), teaching, and consulting. The new Zeno focuses on e-discourses and supports e-moderators in turning discussions into discourses, elaborating the argumentation and carving out rationales.

A discourse is a deliberative, reasoned communication; it is focused and intended to culminate in decision making (Erickson 1999). Turoff et al. (1999) argued that building a discourse grammar, which allows individuals to classify their contributions into meaningful categories, is a collaborative effort and its dynamic evolution is an integral part of the discussion process. A discourse grammar (or ontology) defines labels for contributions, labels for references (directed links) between contributions, and may constrain links with respect to their sources and targets. Supporting communities in evolving their own discourse grammars has been a key issue in the design of Zeno.

4.3.2   Zeno Concepts

As a consequence, Zeno distinguishes three kinds of objects: Sections to tailor the settings for an e-discourse, articles as units of a communication (contributions), and links as directed relations between articles or even sections.

Moderators specify the readers, authors, and co-editors of the section, its discourse grammar, a style sheet to control the presentation, and plugged-in functionality (for mapping, awareness, polling, etc).

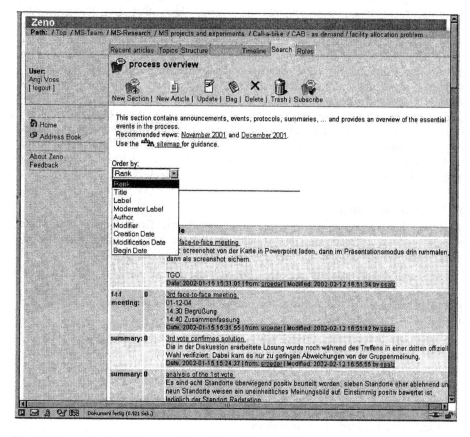

Fig. 6. The search view in the overview section of a spatial decision making discourse in Zeno

An article has a title, usually a note (plain text or html), and possibly document attachments. From its author it may get a label to indicate its pragmatic (or ontological) role in the discourse (e.g. issue, option, criterion, argument, decision, summary, question, comment), and it may receive an additional qualifier from the moderator (e.g. green, yellow, red cards). Articles may be selected (and deselected) as topics and may be ranked to influence their ordering. An article may have temporal references (to be displayed on a timeline), keywords (to be searched together with the title and note), and attributes related to its visibility and accessibility.

Links between articles or sections may be labeled to express relations, such as refers-to, responds-to, justifies, questions, generalizes, suggests, pro, contra) so that complex networks (or hyperthreads) can be built. Links between Zeno articles and sections are visible at both end points and can be traversed in both directions. They are automatically maintained by Zeno, so moderators may edit, copy and move groups of articles with their links.

Zeno links may also point to external web resources; they are used for document references in indigo and for spatial references (to be displayed on a map) in KogiPlan (www.kogiplan.de).

Users are received on a personal home page. Here they can bookmark and subscribe sections in order to be notified of their latest contributions. Each section offers different views: The latest articles, the topics, the complete article structure, a sorted list of articles as a result of a full-text search, the hierarchy of subsections, or the timeline. Authors may create or respond to articles in a section, and moderators may edit, move and copy articles, change links and assign labels, and manipulate sections. Users and groups are administered through an address book.

Zeno can be assessed from any regular web browser without any local installations. The Zeno server is implemented on top of open source products: Tomcat as web server and servlet runner, velocity for templates in the user interface, Java for the kernel, and MySQL for the data base. Zeno itself is available as open source (http://zeno.berlios.de/).

4.3.3   Zeno for indiGo

In Zeno, document-centered discourses, or more specifically, discourses about process models, are made possible through the indiGo integrator and some indigo-specific adaptations of Zeno.

The structure and ordering of process models and their elements is reflected in the hierarchies of sections and their ranking. The mapping between these structures is accomplished through Zeno links, the names of which encode identifiers for the process model and element.

Moderators first create entries for users and groups in the address book. Next, to generate a section for discussing a process, the moderators click on the "discussion" button of the process or any of its elements and then select a group as readers and writers for the discussion. Subsections for discussing process elements are created on demand, when users click on the associated processes and selects the discussion group. The subsections inherit the discourse grammar of their super-section and are restricted to the selected group as authors.

When a user clicks on an "annotation" button for the first time, a personal section is created. This section and its subsections can only be accessed by this user with all rights of a moderator. Subsections for processes and their elements are again created on demand, when the user clicks on the corresponding "annotation" buttons.

The start page of the indiGo system is automatically generated. The upper part displays announcements. These are articles in a section called "StartPage" , can be edited by all indiGo moderators. Beneath the announcements, the start page lists all new articles in the user's discussion groups. This service replaces the subscription and notification mechanism that is otherwise available on the users' personal home page in Zeno.

For the introduction and operational phase of an instantiation of the indiGo Methodology for a certain process model different discourse grammars will be available. "info", "question", "comment", "suggestion", "example" are the article labels during introduction, "observation", "problem", "suggestion", "solution", "example" and "summary" are the article labels during operation. Link labels are in both phases "re", "pro", "con", "see also". Qualifier will include "closed" to indicate threads with a conclusion, and "invalid" to indicate threads that may have become invalid due to modifications of the process model. To come back to the introductory example, Ms Legrelle could have attached a "problem" to the guideline on payment schedules, "re"sponded with a "suggestion" concerning small start-ups, and supported it with a "pro" "example" from the Hydra project.

4.4   CoIN-EF

Compared to the objectives of an organization as captured in its process models, projects have a short-term perspective, oriented towards the goals of the project. Therefore an organizational unit that is responsible for experience management is required and has to be separated from the project teams. As already mentioned, such a separate organizational unit is called experience factory (EF), which for the IESE is operationalized by the CoIN team.

Beside the propagation of knowledge within IESE, CoIN-EF is used as a real-world environment for the development and validation of technologies and methods for goal-oriented EM. Until now IESE has gathered nearly three years of operational experience in maintaining CoIN, and CoIN was successfully transferred to partners and customers, for example in the *IPQM project* for continuous improvement of hospitals in the German healthcare sector (Althoff, Bomarius et al. 1999). Based on these experiences, the requirements of CoIN were widened towards an organization-wide information and knowledge management system.

Within the integrated experience base (EB), all kinds of experience necessary for daily business are stored (e.g., guidelines, or observations). Defined processes populate the EB systematically with experience typically needed by IESE's project teams. The retrieval of experiences from the EB is planned right at the start of the build-up and supports a goal-oriented, context-sensitive, similarity-based retrieval of different kinds of interrelated experiences.

4.4.1   Experiences in CoIN

Within CoIN-EF, lessons learned (LL) about project management are captured. A LL can take on the form of an observation, a problem, guideline, pragmatic solution, or an improvement suggestion. Each LL is personalized to allow a querying IESE member to ask a colleague for further information. The context of these LLs is modeled by the two concepts "project" and "process". A "project" is a characterization of the project where the LL was gained (e.g., person months, duration). The "process" names the business process and thus the project phase in which the LL was gained. Therefore, project team members can specify their current environment as well as the current situation to search the EB for similar experiences.

Observations are facts that are of interest to future projects, often expressing some baseline (e.g., "it took 10% of the total effort to manage the project") or some positive effect (e.g., "the customer was happy because we provided him with a ready-to-use tutorial"). Problems are descriptions of negative situations that occurred during a project (e.g., "the expectations of the customer were not met"). Guidelines, improvement suggestions, and pragmatic solutions relate to one or more problems. Guidelines are recommendations on how a particular business process should be performed. For example, a guideline could be the following: "Interact with the customer frequently, at least twice a month." An improvement suggestion is a proposal to change an artifact to avoid problems that occurred during its usage. Pragmatic solutions are sequences of immediate countermeasures taken by a project team in response to a recognized problem. While a guideline aims at preventing a problem from occurring in the first place, a pragmatic solution is applied after a problem has already occurred.

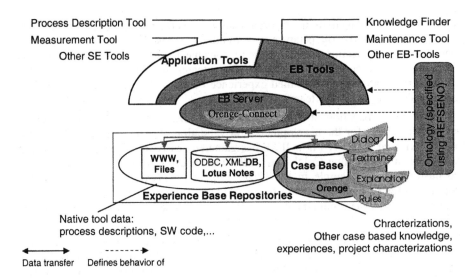

Fig. 7. CoIN's technical infrastructure (INTERESTS)

The technical infrastructure, called INTERESTS (INTElligent REtrieval and STorage System), is shown in Figure 7. It consists of a tool layer for accessing and presenting the EB contents using a standard web browser, a general purpose EB server, and a commercial CBR tool (orenge from empolis, Germany), which is used for the actual EB.

4.4.2   CoIN-EF for indiGo

The integration of CoIN-EF into the indiGo platform will be finished in April 2002. This integration allows to retrieve LLs related to the current process and (project context) by one click. To do so, the current (project) context is specified and stored within the user preferences and is stored persistently across the users sessions.

More challenging will be the integration with tools for knowledge construction: From discourses to experiences and from experiences to process models. As a preparation, the discourse grammar for the operational phase has been designed according to the formats for LLs. This should facilitate a mapping of the articles in a discussion to types of LLs.

4.4.3   Case-Based Reasoning for Sharing Process and Project Knowledge

Since several years there has been a strong tendency in the case-based reasoning (CBR) community (Kolodner 1993) to develop methods for dealing with more complex applications. One example is the use of CBR for knowledge management (KM) (Aha, Becerra-Fernandez et al. 1999). Another one is the integration of CBR with experience factories (Henninger 1995, Althoff & Wilke 1997, Tautz & Althoff 1997, Bergmann, Breen et al. 1999). The latter also contributed to the development of the experience management subfield of KM (Tautz 2000, Bergmann 2001, Althoff, Decker et al. 2001), which already found one implementation through the merger of the German CBR and KM communities (www.experience-management.org, Minor & Staab 2002). Meanwhile many papers have been published that are related to the use of CBR in KM. Weber, Aha, and Becerra-Fernandez (2001) give an overview on intelligent LLs systems, which includes CBR approaches. While Wargitsch (1998) describes how CBR can be used for workflow support, Chen-Burger, Robertson, and Stader (2000) focus on the support for business modeling in general. Decker and Jedlitschka (2001) present a first step how business processes and EM/CBR can be integrated. Further approaches on process-oriented knowledge management and CBR can be found in Weber and Gresse von Wangenheim (2001). CBR-based knowledge reuse for project management is described in Althoff, Nick, and Tautz (1999), Tautz (2000), Brandt and Nick (2001), and Friedrich, Iglezakis et al. (2002). CBR for supporting knowledge mediation is the topic underlying Griffiths, Harrison, and Dearden (1999).

4.5   Text Mining in indiGo

Text mining is concerned with the task of extracting relevant information from natural language text and to search for interesting relationships between the extracted entities. From a linguistic viewpoint natural language exhibits complex structures on different hierarchical levels, which are interconnected to each other (Hrebíček 1996). These structures, however, are tuned to human cognitive abilities. From the perspective of a computational system, which is adopted here, linguistic information appears to be implicitly encoded in an unstructured way and presents a challenge for automatic data processing.

Text classification is one of the basic techniques in the area of text-mining. It means that text documents are filtered into a set of content-categories. For the task of text classification, there are promising approaches, which stand for different learning paradigms, among them, support vector machines (SVM) are one of the most promising solutions (Joachims 1998). AIS has successfully applied SVM to different classification problems - topic detection and author identification (Kindermann, Diederich et al. 2002), multi-class classification (Kindermann, Paaß & Leopold 2001) - on different linguistic corpora: Reuters newswire, English and German newspapers (Leopold & Kindermann 2002), as well as radio-broadcastings (Eickeler, Kindermann et al. 2002). The major problem of applying text classification techniques in the indiGo project is the amount of data. The training of a SVM requires some hundred positive and negative examples for each class to be considered. These data must be collected in the group discussions. The contributions in a discussion group have to annotated with respect to the desired classes by the moderator.

An especially challenging task to text mining systems is to map the unstructured natural text to a structured internal representation (basically a set of data objects). indiGo requires to map text documents generated in the group discussions to structured information of project experiences. However, the limited scope of the indiGo-project - many roles can only be fulfilled by a finite number of subjects (e.g. the number of IESE's employees or costumers is finite) - makes it possible to invent simplifying solutions to many problems, which are not feasible in the general case.

The context of an utterance consists of all elements in a communicative situation that determine the understanding of an utterance in a systematic way. Context divides up into verbal and non-verbal context (Bußmann 1990). Non-verbal context cannot - or at best to a small extent - be conveyed in written text. Abstracting away from the non-verbal context of the situation which a text (spoken or written) is produced, means, that the lost information has to be substituted by linguistic means in order to avoid misunderstandings resulting from the loss of information. This is why spoken and written language differ. Speaker and hearer are exposed to the same contextual situation, which disambiguates their utterances, whereas writer and reader - in the traditional sense of the word - are not.

Computer-mediated communication adopts an intermediate position in this respect. Writer and reader react on each other's utterances as speaker and hearer do. They are in the same communicative situation. But their opportunity to convey non-verbal information is limited as well as the chance to obtain information about the contextual situations of their counterparts.

The context of the communicative situation becomes crucial in the IndiGo setting when discussions are condensed to project experiences. The communicative situation of the discussion is lost and respective information has to be added to the natural language data. This limits the degree of information compaction of linguistic data. Consequently the decontextualization suggested in Figure 1 has to be carefully performed in order to not end up in compressed but nevertheless senseless "structured information". How and to what extent information about the communicative situation can be concentrated or discarded is an interesting research objective of the indiGo project.

To provide the moderator with information about the problem-orientation of the participants in a discussion we propose an "index of speciality of language", which can be calculated on the basis of the agreement of the vocabulary of writer and reader. Self-organizing maps (SOM) (Kohonen 2001) (Merkl 1997) can give an overview over a set of documents, and thus inform the moderator about similar themes that are discussed in different threads. Standard clustering procedures as well the hierarchical analysis of textual similarities (Mehler 2002) can enhance the presentation of textual data in order to support the moderator in formalizing discussion contributions as reusable experiences or cases.

5   Outlook

indiGo was designed to support all kinds of knowledge that have been identified as being import for process learning, namely process models (with their associated templates), experiences from instantiating process models in concrete projects, discussions about processes in closed or open groups, and private annotations of process models. Thus with indiGo, any concerned organization member can make private annotations for a newly introduced, or changed, business process model. Staff can decide which of the issues that attracted their attention should be discussed within a selected group of people. The indiGo technical infrastructure enables the organization of various of such discussion groups based on a customizable discourse grammar, and indiGo's e-moderation method guarantees that such discussions are carried in a structured and goal-oriented manner. This helps to identify valuable experiences, which then are represented as semi-formal cases, and stored in the experience base. Using case-based reasoning, these experiences are then available for both process improvement/change and process execution.

The first version of indiGo was presented in March 2002 at CeBIT. Starting in April 2002, indiGo will be validated within a case study carried out at Fraunhofer IESE in Kaiserslautern, Germany. New project and strategy processes will be introduced for the whole institute and indiGo has been chosen as the process learning platform. We expect very valuable feedback for all the described indiGo methods and technologies.

In parallel, specified but not yet implemented features will be realized. For instance, if a process model is modified or reorganized, the corresponding annotations and discussions should automatically be marked for re-validation or be reorganized accordingly. In parallel, the indiGo platform will be extended to include the components on the lower level in Figure 3, starting with CoIN-EF.

As soon as discussions will become available from the case study, text mining experiments can begin. For that purpose, the discussions in Zeno will be exported in GXL, an XML dialect for graph structures. Private annotations remain private and will not be subject to text mining.

Beyond the current project we consider the possibility to extend the indiGo approach to applications where process models do not play such a central role. Although a platform for organizational learning should eventually cover all knowledge categories treated in indiGo, the first steps to organizational learning need not necessarily involve process models. Maybe, an organization would first like to invest into an experience base or into a communication platform, and add process models only later. The challenging research question here is, to which degree indiGo's methods and technologies can still be applied or easily tailored to such an organization's needs.

References

Aha, D.W., Becerra-Fernandez, I., Maurer, F., and Muñoz-Avila, H. (Eds.) (1999). Exploring Synergies of Knowledge Management and Case-Based Reasoning: Papers from the AAAI 1999 Workshop (Technical Report WS-99-10). Menlo Park, CA: AAAI Press.

Althoff, K.-D., Birk, A., Hartkopf, S., Müller, W., Nick, M., Surmann, D. & Tautz, C. (1999) Managing Software Engineering Experience for Comprehensive Reuse; Proceedings of the Eleventh Conference on Software Engineering and Knowledge Engineering, Kaiserslautern, Germany, June 1999; Knowledge Systems Institute; Skokie, Illinois, USA.

Althoff, K.-D., Bomarius, F., Müller, W. & Nick, M. (1999). Using a Case-Based Reasoning for Supporting Continuous Improvement Processes. In: P. Perner (ed.), *Proc. German Workshop on Machine Learning*, Technical Report, Institute for Image Processing and Applied Informatics, Leipzig, 8 pages.

Althoff, K.-D., Decker, B., Hartkopf, S., Jedlitschka, A., Nick, M. & Rech, J. (2001). Experience Management: The Fraunhofer IESE Experience Factory. In P. Perner (ed.), Proc. Industrial Conference Data Mining, Leipzig, 24.-25. Juli 2001, Institut für Bildverarbeitung und angewandte Informatik

Althoff, K.-D., Feldmann, R. & Müller, W. (eds.) (2001). *Advances in Learning Software Organizations*. Springer Verlag, LNCS 2176, September 2001.

Althoff, K.-D., Nick, M. & Tautz, C. (1999). An Application Implementing Reuse Concepts of the Experience Factory for the Transfer of CBR System Know-How. In: E. Melis (ed.), *Proc. of the Seventh German Workshop on Case-Based Reasoning (GWCBR'99)*.

Althoff, K.-D. & Wilke, W. (1997). Potential Uses of Case-Based Reasoning in Experience Based Construction of Software Systems and Business Process Support. In: R. Bergmann & W. Wilke (eds.), *Proc. of the 5th German Workshop on Case-Based Reasoning*, LSA-97-01E, Centre for Learning Systems and Applications, University of Kaiserslautern, 31-38.

Bandinelli, S., Fuggetta, A., Lavazza, L., Loi, M. & Picco G.P. (1995). Modeling and improving an industrial software process, Transactions on Software Engineering, 440-454.

Basili, V.R., Caldiera, G., Rombach, D. (1994). Experience Factory; In Marciniak, J.J. ed., Encyclopedia of Software Engineering, vol 1, 469–476; John Wiley & Sons.

Becker-Kornstaedt, U. (2001). Towards Systematic Knowledge Elicitation for Descriptive Software Process Modeling. In Frank Bomarius and Seija Komi-Sirviö, editors, Proceedings of the Third International Conference on Product-Focused Software Processes Improvement (PROFES), Lecture Notes in Computer Science 2188, pages 312-325, Kaiserslautern, September 2001. Springer.

Becker-Kornstaedt, U. & Belau, W. (2000). Descriptive Process Modeling in an Industrial Environment: Experience and Guidelines. In R. Conradi, editor, *Proceedings of the 7th European Workshop on Software Process Technology (EWSPT 7)*, Kaprun, Austria, pages 177–189, Lecture Notes in Computer Sciences, Springer-Verlag. 2000.

Becker-Kornstaedt, U., Hamann, D., Kempkens, R., Rösch, P., Verlage, M., Webby, R., & Zettel, J. (1999). Support for the Process Engineer: The Spearmint Approach to Software Process Definition and Process Guidance. In Proceedings of the 11th Conference on Advanced Information Systems Engineering (CAISE '99), Heidelberg, Germany, June 1999. Lecture Notes on Computer Science, Springer-Verlag.

Becker-Kornstaedt, U. & Verlage, M. (1999). The V-Model Guide: Experience with a Web-based Approach for Process Support; Proceedings of Software Technology and Engineering Practice (STEP).

Bergmann, R. (2001). Experience management - foundations, development methodology, and internet-based applications. Postdoctoral thesis, Department of Computer Science, University of Kaiserslautern (submitted).

Bergmann, R., Breen, S., Göker, M., Manago, M. & Wess, S. (1999). *Developing Industrial CBR Applications. The INRECA-Methodology*. Springer Verlag, LNAI 1612.

Brandt, M. & Nick, M. (2001). Computer-Supported Reuse of Project Management Experience with an Experience Base. In *Althoff, Feldemann & Müller (2001)*, 178-191.

Bröckers, A., Lott, C.M., Rombach, H. D. & Verlage, M. (1995). MVP-L Language Report Version 2; Technical Report University of Kaiserslautern, Department of Computer Science 265 / 95.

Bußmann, Hadumod (1990): Lexikon der Sprachwissenschaft, Kröner: Stuttgart.

Conklin, J. and M. Begeman (1988) "gIBIS: A Hypertext Tool for Exploratory Policy Discussion", *Transactions of Office Information Systems*, 6(4): 303-331.

Curtis, B., Kellner, M. I. & Over, J. (1992). Process Modeling. *Communications of the ACM.*

Decker, B. & Jedlitschka, A. (2001). The Integrated Corporate Information Network iCoIN: A Comprehensive Web-Based Experience Factory. In *Althoff, Feldmann & Müller (2001)*, 192-206.

Dellen, B., Könnecker, A. & Scott, L. (2000). *Process Modeling Tool Evaluation.* IESE-Report 002.00/E, Fraunhofer IESE, Kaiserslautern, Germany.

Eickeler, Stefan & Kindermann, Jörg & Larson, Martha & Leopold, Edda & Paaß, Gerhard: Classification of Spoken Documents using SVM and Sub-word Units; submitted to Neurocomputing, Special Issue on Support Vector Machines.

Erickson, T. (1999): "Persistent Conversation. An introduction". Journal of Computer-Mediated Communication, 4.

Raimund L. Feldmann, Michael Frey, Marco Habetz, and Manoel Mendonca (2000). Applying Roles in Reuse Repositories. In Proceedings of the Twelfth Conference on Software Engineering and Knowledge Engineering, Kaiserslautern, Germany, July 2000. Knowledge Systems Institute, Skokie, Illinois, USA.

Friedrich, R., Iglezakis, I., Klein, W. & Pregizer, S. (2002). Experience-based decision support for project management with case-based reasoning.. In Minor & Staab (2002), 139-150.

Gordon, Thomas F., und Nikos Karacapilidis. 1997. "The Zeno Argumentation Framework." Pp. 10-18 in *Proceedings of the Sixth International Conference on Artificial Intelligence and Law.*

Griffiths, A.D., Harrison, M.D. & Dearden, A.M. (1999). Case Based Reasoning Systems for Knowledge Mediation. in M. A. Sasse and C. Johnson (eds.), *Proceedings of Interact 99,* (Edinburgh), IOS Press. pp. 425-433.

Henninger, S. (1995). Developing Domain Knowledge Through the Reuse of Project Experiences. *Proc. Symposium on Software Reusability (SSR '95), Seattle WA, April 1995.*

Hřebíccek, Luděk & Altmann, Gabriel(1996): The Levels of Order in Language, Glottometrika 15, 38-61.

Joachims, T. (1998). Text categorization with Support Vector Machines: Learning with many relevant features.Proc 10th European Conference on Machine Learning (ECML 98), LNCS 1398, Springer Verlag, pp137-142

Kellner, M. I., Becker-Kornstaedt, U., Riddle, W. E., Tomal, J. & Verlage, M. (1998). Process Guides: Effective Guidance for Process Participants. In *Proceedings of the Fifth International Conference on the Software Process*, pages 11-25, Chicago, IL, USA, June 1998. ISPA Press.

Kindermann, Jörg & Paaß, Gerhard & Leopold, Edda (2001): *Error Correcting Codes with Optimized Kullback-Leibler Distances for Text Categorization*; PKDD'01; 3 - 7 September 2001 in Freiburg.

Kindermann, Jörg & Diederich, Joachim & Leopold, Edda & Paaß, Gerhard: *Identifying the Author of a Text with Support Vector Machines*; accepted at *Applied Intelligence.*

Kohonen, Teuvo (2001): Self-organizing maps, Springer: Berlin, Heidelberg, New York

Kolodner, J. L. (1993). *Case-Based Reasoning.* Morgan Kaufmann.

Kunz, Werner und Horst W.J. Rittel (1970): "Issues as elements of information systems." Center for Planning and Development Research, Institute of Urban and Regional Development Research. Working Paper 131, University of California, Berkeley.

Leopold, Edda & Kindermann, Jörg (2002): *Text Categorization with Support Vector Machines. How to Represent Texts in Input Space?;* in: *Machine Learning* 46, 423 - 444.

Märker, O., Hagedorn, H., Trénel, M. and Gordon, T. F. 2002 'Internet-based Citizen Participation in the City of Esslingen. Relevance - Moderation - Software', in M. Schrenk (ed) CORP 2002 - "Who plans Europe's future?" Wien: Selbstverlag des Instituts für EDV-gestützte Methoden in Architektur und Raumplanung der Technischen Universität Wien.

Maurer, F. & Holz, H. (1999). Process-Oriented Knowledge Management For Learning Software Organizations, Proceedings of 12th Knowledge Acquisition For Knowledge-Based Systems Workshop 1999 (KAW99); Banff, Canada.

Mehler, Alexander (2002): Hierarchical analysis of text similarity data, in: Thorsten Joachims & Edda Leopold (eds.): Künstliche Intelligenz, Schwerpunkt Textmining, to appear.

Merkl, Dieter (1997): Exploration of Document Collections with Self-Organizing Maps: A Novel Approach to Similarity Representation, *a novel approach to similarity visualization"*. Proceedings of the European Symposium on Principles of Data Mining and Knowledge Discovery (PKDD'97), (Trondheim, Norway. June).

Minor, M. & Staab, S. (eds.) (2002). 1st German Workshop on Experience management – Sharing Experiences about the Sharing of Experience, Berlin, March 7-8, 2002, Lecture Notes in Informatics, Gesellschaft für Informatik (Bonn).

Osterweil, L. (1987). Software Processes Are Software Too, Association for Computer Machinery (ACM).

Scheer, A.W. (1997). Referenzmodelle für industrielle Geschäftsprozesse (siebte Auflage), Springer Verlag.

Scott L, Jeffery D.R., Becker-Kornstaedt U. (2001). Preliminary Results of an Industrial EPG Evaluation. In F.Maurer; B. Dellen; J. Grundy; B. Koetting (eds.), Proc. 4th ICSE Workshop on Software Engineering over the Internet, Toronto Canada, 12-19 May. 2001, IEEE Computer Society, California, USA, pp55-58.

Sumner, T. & Buckingham Shum, S. (1998) "From Documents to Discourse: Shifting Conceptions of Scholarly Publishing", Proc. CHI 98: Human Factors in Computing Systems, 18-23 April, 1998, Los Angeles, CA. ACM Press: New York

Tautz, C. (2000). *Customizing Software Engineering Experience Management Systems to Organizational Needs.* Doctoral Dissertation, Department of Computer Science, University of Kaiserslautern, Germany.

Tautz, C. & Althoff, K.-D. (1997). Using Case-Based Reasoning for Reusing Software Knowledge. *Case-Based Reasoning Research and Development – Second International Conference (ICCBR97),* Providence, RI, Springer Verlag.

Turoff, M., Hiltz, S. R., Bieber, M., Fjermestadt, J. and Ajaz, R. (1999): "Collaborative discourse structures in computer-mediated group communications". Journal of Computer-Mediated Communication, 4.

von Hunnius, J.-P. (2000). WESPI – Web Supported Process Improvement. In K.-D. Althoff & W. Müller (eds.), Proc. 2nd Internationl Workshop on Learning Software Organizations, June 20, 2000, Oulu Finland, Fraunhofer IESE, Kaiserslautern, Germany.

Voss, A. (to appear (2002)): „Zeno – Software für Online-Diskurse in der Mediation". In Online-Mediation. Theorie und Praxis computer-unterstützter Konfliktmittlung(Eds, Märker, O. and Trenél, M.) Sigma, Berlin.

Voss, A., Roeder, S. and Wacker, U. (to appear (2002)): „IT-support for mediation in decision making - A role playing experiment". In Online-Mediation. Theorie und Praxis computer-unterstützter Konfliktmittlung.(Eds, Märker, O. and Trenél, M.) Sigma, Berlin.

Wargitsch, C. (1998). *Ein Beitrag zur Integration von Workflow- und Wissensmanagement unter besonderer Berücksichtigung komplexer Geschäftsprozesse.* Doctoral Dissertation, University of Erlangen-Nürnberg, Germany.

Weber, R., Aha, D.W., & Becerra-Fernandez, I. (2001). Intelligent lessons learned systems. Expert Systems with Applications, 20, 17-34.

Weber, R. & Gresse von Wangenheim, C. (eds.) (2001). Proceedings of the Workshop Program at the Fourth International Conference on Case-Based Reasoning, Technical Note AIC-01-003, Washington, DC: Naval Reasearch Laboratory, Naval Research Center for Applied Research in Artificial Intelligence.

Workflow Management Facility Specification (2000). V1.2, Object Management Group; http://www.omg.org/.

Yun-Heh Chen-Burger, Dave Robertson & Jussi Stader (2000). A Case-Based Reasoning Framework for Enterprise Model Building, Sharing and Reusing. *Proc. ECAI 2000 Workshop on Knowledge Management and Organizational Memories*, Berlin.

Genomic Data Explosion – The Challenge for Bioinformatics?

Änne Glass and Thomas Karopka

University of Rostock, Institute for Medical Informatics and Biometry,
Rembrandt-Str. 16/17, 18055 Rostock, Germany
{aenne.glass,thomas.karopka}@medizin.uni-rostock.de
http://www.med.uni-rostock.de

Abstract. A dramatic increase in the amount of genomic expression data with knowledge in to mine for getting a principal understanding of "what is a considered disease at the genomic level" is available today. We give a short overview about common processing of micro array expression data. Furthermore we introduce a complex bioinformatic approach[1] combining properly several analyzing methods to mine gene expression data and biomedical literature. Gene patterns and gene relation information as results from data and text mining is to be considered as integral part for modeling genetic networks. We apply methods of case-based-reasoning for generating a similarity tree consisting of genetic networks. These networks are efficient facilities to understand the dynamic of pathogenic processes and to answer a question like "what is a disease x in the genomic sense"?

1 Introduction

A dramatic increase in the amount of electronic stored information has been seen in recent years. It has been estimated that the amount of information in the world doubles every 20 month. These new data promise to enhance fundamental understanding of life on the molecular level [1]. The advent of new technologies has empowered genome researchers to measure the concentrations of every transcript in the cell in a single experiment. It has added new dimensions to our ability to leverage information from genome sequencing projects into a more comprehensive and holistic understanding of cell physiology. The scientific community has not determined how to cope with the massive amounts of data explored and interpreted in the context of other sources of biological and medical knowledge. For example, at Stanford and Rosetta alone, more than 30 million independent gene expression measurements (one gene, one condition) have been made between 1997 and 1999 [2]. The way we do biology changes towards a more holistic view of biological systems which is significantly different from the classical idea of investigating one or a few genes at a time.

---

[1] Funded by German Ministry for Education and Research (Bundesministerium für Bildung und Forschung, BMBF); Grant Number: FKZ 01GG9831

P. Perner (Ed.): Advances in Data Mining 2002, LNAI 2394, pp. 80-98, 2002.

A great intellectual challenge in using new technologies is devising a way in which to extract the full meaning of the data stored in large experimental gene expression datasets. As "data mining" has been defined as "the exploration and analysis, by automatic or semi-automatic methods, of large quantities of data in order to discover meaningful patterns and rules" [3]. In brief, the goal is to convert data into information and then information into knowledge [4]. Freeing this knowledge is the key to increase performance and success in the information age. Exactly this task is a key challenge for bioinformatics. With the acceptance of a challenge of such a complexity it is clear that also the solution to be provided by bioinformatics will be very complex.

In this paper we want to address the complexity of this bioinformatic demand and discuss some of the technical and intellectual issues involved in these processes, describe some of the ways in which they are currently being addressed. We want to introduce a bioinformatic approach combining experimental micro array data with several methods such as database techniques, data mining, artificial intelligence, statistics, modeling and computer graphics as shown in Fig 1. It is not done to use this or that special method or to find the right one! The point is that by coupling several proper methods in a well working bioinformatic software system it is expected to achieve synergetic effects. Fig. 1 shows a proper combination of several methods of different scientific domains to solve the complex task described above. Basic components of such a complex bioinformatic working facility are a central data storage and tools for analyzing and presenting data and results.

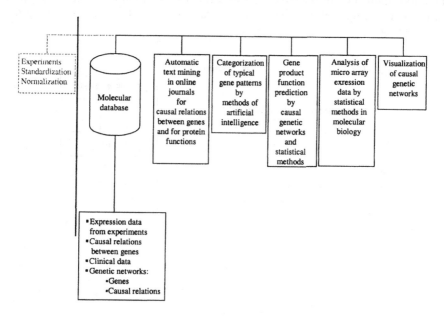

Fig. 1. Genome oriented bioinformatics at the Institute for Medical Informatics and Biometry, University of Rostock

A molecular database stores micro array expression data from experiments in a standardized and normalized form as well as deliverables from other system components and clinical patient data available in a coded form from medical faculty. Clinical data are an essential "background" for effective analyzing expression data.

Deliverables from automatic text mining tool are information about causal relations between genes obtained from online journals of biomedical literature. AI-methods like neural networks can provide categories of gene patterns which are typical in a general sense for a considered disease. Results of the latter both methods are integral parts of genetic networks which are modeled as a primary objective of the bioinformatic system. With the help of models we have made incredible progress in deciphering what we know today about dynamic cell. A visualization tool is utilized for graphical presentation of genetic networks. Based on genomic data analysis and genetic networks as models we want to give a bioinformatic approach for understanding the dynamic of pathogenic processes and to answer questions like "what is a disease x in the genomic sense"?

2 Micro Array Expression Data – Results from Wet Lab and Data Analysis

2.1 Lab Phase

The information flow in processing micro array data is primarily based on samples and micro arrays for making hybridization in laboratories. All this occurs during the lab phase (Fig. 2).

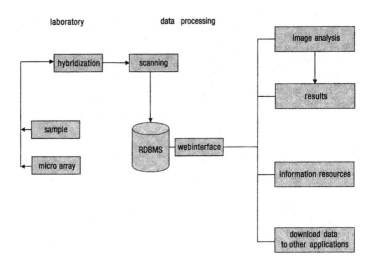

Fig. 2. Information flow in processing micro arrays

cDNA micro arrays are capable of profiling gene expression patterns of tens of thousands of genes in a single experiment. DNA targets are arrayed onto glass slides or membranes and probed with fluorescent- or radioactively-labelled cDNA [5]. Interesting is the image analysis and data extraction. The highly regular arrangement of detector elements and crisply delineated signals that result from robotic printing and confocal imaging of detected arrays renders image data amenable to extraction by highly developed, digital image processing procedures. Mathematical morphology methods can be used to predict the likely shape and placement of the hybridization signal. In contrast, extraction of data from film or phosphor-image representations of radioactive hybridisations presents many difficulties for image analysis.

2.2 Data Processing Phase

Data processing starts with the phase of digitalizing (Fig. 2). A scanner is used for digitalizing arrays. Digital data are stored in a database - a central part of the whole laboratory information management system (LIMS) which manages hybridization results in general. All array methods require the construction of databases within a LIMS for the management of information on the genes represented on the array, the primary results of hybridization and the construction of algorithms to examine the outputs of single or multiple array experiments.

Data analysis in this phase is often based on correlation methods developed for the analysis of data which is more highly constrained than at the transcript level.

Scanning and image processing are currently resource-intensive tasks, requiring to ensure that grids are properly aligned. Artefacts have to be labelled and properly excluded from analysis. Standard input and output formats have to be fixed, automation of identifying features and artefacts have to be made sure. Providing routine quality assessment and the assignment of robust confidence statistics of gene expression data is not simple. The quality assurance information should be transmitted with the primary data.The basic idea is to reduce an image of spots of varying intensities into a table with a measure of the intensity for each spot. There is as yet no common manner of extracting this information, and many scientists are still writing customized software for this purpose. A variety of software tools have been developed for use in analysing micro array data and processing array images [6]. Some tools for analysing micro array data are available at http://genome-www5.stanford.edu/MicroArray/SMD/restech.html. This software is provided by micro arraying groups from Stanford. Especially a tool for processing fluorescent images of micro arrays called ScanAlyze is provided for free download.

Technologies for whole-genome RNA expression studies are becoming increasingly reliable and accessible. Universal standards to make the data more suitable for comparative analysis and for inter-operability with other information resources have been yet to emerge [2]. In carrying out comparisons of expression data using measurements from a single array or multiple arrays, the question of normalizing data arises. There are essentially two strategies that can be followed in carrying out the normalization: to consider all of the genes in the sample or to designate a subset expected to be unchanging over most circumstances. In either case, variance of the normalization set can be used to generate estimates of expected variance, leading to predict confidence intervals. A lot of explicit methods have been developed which make use of a subset of genes for normalization, and extract from the variance of this subset statistics for evaluating the significance of observed changes in the complete dataset [7].

Executable investigation levels of gene data analysis are genome, transcriptome, proteome and metabolome. The last three levels can be distinguished from the first one by context dependence. The entire complement of mRNA molecules, proteins or metabolites in an organism, organ or tissue varies with it's physiological, pathological or developmental condition. The analysis of transcriptome using mRNA expression data is providing amounts of data about gene function, but it is an indirect approach because mRNA are transmitters of genetic information, not functional cellular entities. Comprehensive analysis of proteins and metabolites are more technical demanding [8]. A summary for minimum information about a micro array experiment (MIAME) now available in version 1.1 is developed by the object management group (OMG). This standard gives the minimum information required to unambiguously interpret and potentially verify array based gene expression monitoring experiments. MIAME aims to define the core that is common to most experiments and is a set of guidelines. A standard micro array data model and exchange format (MAGE) has been recently developed by the OMG [9]. MIAME is used for standardizing our data from micro array expression experiments.

To speed up the exploitation of human genome sequencing efforts, the European Bioinformatics Institute (EBI) – an outstation of the European Molecular Biology Laboratory (EMBL) – is launching a publicly accessible repository for DNA micro array-based gene expression data. ArrayExpress, a public database (http://www.ebi.ac.uk/microarray/ArrayExpress/arrayexpress.html) for micro array based gene expression data, supports all the requirements specified by the MIAME and aims to store MIAME compliant data. This database will allow to cross-validate data obtained by different technologies.

2.3 Data Analysis

A variety of techniques has established to monitor the abundance for all of an organism's genes [10], [11], [12]. Some of them should be considered:

Average Difference (Avg Diff) – a Parameter Used for Analyzing Expression Data. As we use the technology of Affymetrix™ (glass slides, fluorescent-labelled cDNA) we want to introduce one of the resulting analysis parameters of data processing which includes information about fluorescence intensity – the average difference. This parameter can be interpreted as a gene expression value at mRNA level. That is the reason why this parameter is often used for data analysis of expression experiments. But if we look at this parameter in detail we will find, that there are some points to be noticed. Observing the statistical distribution of this parameter we will note that there are no values in the range of (-1, +1). The sector around null is not specified by the system. Furthermore we found an unsymmetrical distribution comparing two nearly identical expression experiments. The outcome of this is the question whether this is a systematic error based on two independent analysing algorithms for the positive and negative range or maybe the data processing method is extremely sensitive to minimal influences. At least these points are to be kept in mind when using the avg diff - and only this parameter - for getting analysing results of gene expression data. A practicable example for using the avg diff by integrating into the expression data analysis is given by [13]. Gene expression analysis of oligo nucleotide micro arrays to determine gene expression profiles of the inflamed spinal cords of experimental autoimmune encephalomyelitis (EAE) mice at the onset and at the peak of the disease are described. Of the approximately 11 000 genes studied, 213 were regulated differentially and 100 showed consistent differential regulation throughout the disease. These results are obtained using among others the avg diff and several clustering methods in the data processing phase.

Graphical Plot – often Called Clustering. A feature of gene expression is the tendency of expression data to organize genes into functional categories. It is not very surprising that genes that are expressed together are sharing common functions. So we can cluster genes if they are expressed with the same expression profile under same conditions. But what is that – clustering genes? And how to do that right? We find the word clustering nearly in every publication about micro array data analysis. Often this word is used in a very common context, e.g. grouping genes by their expression level or by any other parameter they are labelled with. View the expression profile under specified experimental conditions or under time. Independent of whether the data sets originate from drug responses, molecular anatomy studies or disease models, any analysis starts with a grouping of expression patterns according to their similarity and existing annotations. So the next challenge in expression analysis lies in comparing diverse data sets for which it would not make sense to analyse per cluster analysis the data together *a priori*. Graphical tools can help here to illustrate more-complex relationships. Often is meant a kind of grouping (clustering) with a graphical approach. The result will be a graphical presentation of similar profiles in time, space or under special experimental conditions like concentration gradient.

Cluster Analysis. As described above we will find several approaches of grouping (clustering) data, but it is a difference whether making a clustering which means a graphical grouping or a clustering which means cluster analysis, actually coming from the field of multivariate statistics. The term "clustering" is applied in both contexts. But the idea in the latter case is to process a cluster analysis. This is an exact defined statistical domain with several methods to be practised. Cluster analysis is a set of methods for constructing a (hopefully) sensible and informative classification of an initially unclassified set of data, using the variable values observed on each individual [14]. Given a sample of genes with an expression value we are looking for a characterization of potential clusters of genes and a state which gene is to be assigned to which cluster. We will get a result of statistical analysing algorithm. This could be a cluster schedule in form of a table or list of all genes according each to a cluster number and an according coefficient which gives a value for the distance to the next (nearest) cluster. In most cases there is also given a graphical plot, a dendrogram in case of hierarchical cluster analysis e.g. A very efficient software which performs both variants of "clustering" – various graphical approaches and cluster analysis tools too – is for example the GeneSpring software by Silicon Genetics available at http://www.sigenetics.com/cgi/SiG.cgi/index.smf.

Another system for processing cluster analysis of genome-wide expression data from DNA micro array hybridization is described in [4]. This system uses standard statistical algorithms to arrange genes according to similarity in pattern of gene expression. Although various clustering methods can usefully organize tables of gene expression measurements, the resulting ordered but still massive collection of numbers remains difficult to assimilate. Therefore it is useful to combine clustering methods with graphical representation of the primary data. And to give in this way the scientists a representation of complex gene expression data that, through statistical organization and graphical display, allows them to assimilate and explore the data in a natural intuitive manner.

Principal Component Analyses (PCA). One of the most complex multivariate methods of statistics is PCA, which preferably allows to simplify high-complex data records by reduction of dimensions. In this sense it is a useful mathematical framework for processing expression data. But this approach leads to difficulties in the interpretation of the results. The fact is known in general, but it complicates itself just within a brand new and high-complex research context such as the field of genomics. Nevertheless scientists from Stanford e.g. describe a method for singular value decomposition (SVD) in transforming genome-wide expression data from genes x arrays space to reduced space for processing and modelling [1].

Correlations between Genes. And last but not least there is often spoken about correlations in the context of gene expression analysis. Correlation is a general term for independence between pairs of variables [14]. Therewith is often meant a look at the scatter plot of for instance two experiments to detect something like a cigar in the plot which means the genes seem to be linear correlated in their expression. This is a kind of preliminary investigation to proceed a correlation analysis proving the existence of a correlation. A metric is to develop describing the similarity of two genes over a series of conditions. This could be a proper correlation coefficient as Pearson or Kendall e.g. as an index that quantifies the linear relationship between a pair of variables. And furthermore this coefficient can be tested under distribution assumptions. The coefficient takes values between [−1, +1], with the sign indicating the direction of the relationship and the numerical magnitude its strength. Values of − 1 or 1 indicate that the sample values fall on a straight line. A value of zero indicates the lack of any linear relationship between two variables. So the result will give a proposition about the existence of the hypothetical correlation. Or better said: at the best the result will be a proof that there is not no correlation existing. And to come to end: whether this proved correlation is indeed a causal one as wanted - this is something else.

In this paragraph we gave a short overview about several mostly statistical methods usually applied to mine genomic expression data. In the next paragraph we will introduce a whole software system architecture which is able to perform modelling of genetic networks using the results from micro array expression data analysis.

3 A System Architecture for Mining Micro Array Expression Data

Mining genomic data obtained in the labs of physicians or biologists is a research task from high topicality. But as well frequently are found applications in which text information from journals as results from lab data mining should be mined in turn. In this context we find often applications of methods like parsing documents of text for special words or phrases, methods like information retrieval as a collection of data and information, methods like information extraction to convert no-structured text into structures for storing it into a database.

But it is not done with mining information and put them into a structured form for a database storing. Our intention goes still a step further: we want to mine data with the aim of using the mined information to built up models. The results of data mining should be our input for modelling genetic networks automatically. These networks should characterize diseases at a genomic level. The transcript level could provide new perspectives on the operation of genetic networks [5]. Comparisons of expression profiles will undoubtedly provide useful insights into the molecular pathogenesis of a variety of diseases [15], [16]. And this is the point when data mining results into knowledge in fact. A bioinformatic software system architecture which is aimed to perform this by practicing the import and analysis of genomic expression data for generating and presenting genetic networks is shown in Fig. 3.

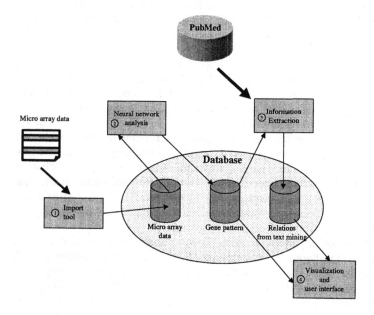

Fig. 3. The architecture of a bioinformatic software system for mining micro array expression data

Main components of the system are 1) an import tool for gene expression micro array data, 2) an expression data analyzing tool using AI-methods, 3) a tool for automatic mining causal gene relation information from public internet databases, and 4) a visualization tool for presenting genetic networks [17]. Gene expression data are provided by different university research groups. Data are validated from technical errors and standardized for import into the software system by a pre-import filter tool written on Excel Visual Basic Application (VBA) which is working directly on lab exported micro array expression data. In the next paragraphs we describe in detail, how such an architecture will perform the data processing part. Especially on 3) we will come more in detail.

4 Modeling Genetic Networks

4.1 Why Modeling?

Most of diseases are caused by a set of gene defects, which occur in a complex association. The association scheme of expressed genes can be modelled by genetic networks. The key is to keep things simple, at least to start with [18]. Just measuring levels of mRNA tells scientists that a gene has been activated, but does not detail the amount of protein it encodes, or which task that protein fulfils in cell dynamic. The future will be the study of the genes and proteins of organisms in the context of their informational networks. Scientists from independent Institute for Systems Biology (ISB) plan to produce a complete mathematical description of complex biological systems e.g. the immune system and complex conditions such as cancer or heart disease. All these efforts will culminate in the assembling of the biological equivalent of a virtual cell. Genetic networks are efficient facilities to understand the dynamic of pathogenic processes by modelling molecular reality of cell conditions.

Genetic networks consists of first, a set of genes of specified cells, tissues or species and second, causal relations between these genes determining the functional condition of the biological system, i.e. under disease. A relation between two genes will exist if they both are directly or indirectly associated with disease. Our goal is to characterize diseases - especially autoimmune diseases like chronic pancreatitis (CP), multiple sclerosis (MS), rheumatoid arthritis (RA) - by genetic networks generated by a computer system. We want to introduce this practice as a bioinformatic approach for finding targets.

Genes that follow similar patterns of expression are likely to share common molecular control processes. Furthermore, assuming that there is a reason for these genes to be expressed together, it is possible that they participate in a similar or complementary set of functions required by the organism under a given condition [19]. Comparison of expression profiles will not deliver the kind of intimate understanding of the highly inter-related control circuitry that is necessary to achieve true understanding of genome function [5]. But with an optimal composition of expression profile analysis methods mentioned above combined with modelling we will get a powerful instrument to describe diseases in a highly abstract way. So we have to combine the library of tools we use to analyse expression data – recruiting as well statisticians and mathematicians as biologists and physicians to consider multi variant problems of a never knowing size and complexity. In the next few paragraphs methods are discussed which we want to combine for generating genetic networks.

4.2 Processing an Artificial Neural Network to Classify Gene Expression Patterns

An artificial neural network is utilized for classifying diseases to specific diagnostic categories based on their gene expression signatures. We chose a neural network of adaptive resonance theory (ART). An ART net works like a self-organizing neural pattern recognition machine. The five major properties of the ART system are plasticity as well as stability, furthermore sensitivity to novelty, attentional mechanisms and complexity. The network architecture of type ART1 self-organises and self-stabilises its recognition codes and categorises arbitrarily many and arbitrarily complex binary input patterns [20]. We obtain the input patterns for ART1 from gene expression micro array data of different samples of the same disease by using binary coding. As result of ART1 analysis we get a specific pattern of together expressed genes, which shall be deemed to be typical in general for a considered disease. Such a resulting gene pattern is one of the integral parts essential necessary for generating genetic networks.

By the way there are other interesting bioinformatic applications of neural networks discussed in the biomedical literature as for instance an approach for classifying nursing care needed, using incomplete data [21], for detecting periodicities in the protein sequence and increasing in this way the prediction accuracy of secondary structure [22] or predicting drug absorption using structural properties [23].

4.3 Text Mining

Mining Causal Relationship between Genes from Unstructured Text. Using the method described in 5.2. a subset of genes is classified by the neural network for a special biological context, e.g. for a considered disease. As we want to automatically construct a causal genetic network, the next type of information we need concerns causal relationships between classified genes.

One of the richest sources of knowledge nowadays is the internet. This is especially true for the biological domain and within this domain for the field of genomics. A huge amount of data is now available to the public. Much of this data is stored in publicly available databases. Therefore it is reasonable to integrate this knowledge into the construction of genetic networks. A straight forward approach is to find databases which contain the type of information we are looking for. For our work we found the appropriate information in the GeNet database. We designed and implemented a tool that consists of three sequential working components: first a database adapter that connects to the internet database GeNet, queries the data and stores all query results locally on the computer. A parser tool analyses the stored data and extracts the wanted information. In the last step a filter tool searches for data redundancy and inconsistency and prepares resulting data with gene relation information for import into the software system for generating and presenting genetic networks.

But a lot of specific knowledge is not available in such a structured form. It is distributed somewhere in the net and it is presented in unstructured text. In our case relationships between genes are not available in special databases but it may be found in the biomedical literature. Most of these articles are available online. One of the key databases for publications in this field is the PubMed database. PubMed contains over 11 million abstracts today and approximately 40,000 new abstracts are added each month. To use this source of information we have to deploy more sophisticated methods than those described above. One way to integrate this knowledge into the analysing process of the micro array data automatically is the usage of techniques of Information Extraction (IE). In this paragraph we first give a definition of IE. Than we will focus on the problems to deal with when applying IE to the biological domain. Further we give an overview of related work in this field and finally we describe the design of the IE module in our system.

IE is a relatively new discipline within the more general field of Natural Language Processing (NLP). IE is not Information Retrieval (IR), in which key words are used to select relevant documents from a large collection e.g. the internet. In contrast IE extracts relevant information from documents and can be used to post-process the IR output. As usual with emerging technologies, there are a number of definitions of information extraction. We understand IE as a *procedure that selects, extracts and combines data from unstructured text in order to produce structured information.* This structured information can than be easily transformed to a database record.

Much of the work in this field is influenced by the Message Understanding Conferences (MUCs) instituted by the Defence Advanced Research Projects Agency (DARPA) in the late '80s. The MUCs were created to have a platform for the evaluation of IE systems. For this purpose a set of 5 tasks described further below were defined which the competing systems have to fulfil. Altogether 7 Conferences were held, each with a different focus and additional tasks defined. MUC-7 was concerned with newspaper articles about space vehicle and missile launches. The defined tasks were also adopted more or less in most of the IE systems implemented in other domains than specified by MUC-7. The tasks can be defined as follows:

- Named entity recognition   (NE),
  The NE task deals with the identification of predefined entities (e.g. names, organizations, locations etc.). In our case these entities are gene or protein names.
- Coreference resolution   (CO),
  This task requires connecting all references to "identical" entities. This includes variant forms of name expressions (e.g. Paul/ he/…)
- Template Element Filling   (TE),
  The required information should be extracted from the text an filled into predefined templates which reflect a structured representation of the information wanted.
- Template Relations   (TR),
  TR covers identifying relationships between template elements.
- Scenario Template   (ST).
  The ST task fits TE and TR results into specified event scenarios.

A more detailed description of the tasks may be found in the MUCs Proceedings (http://www.itl.nist.gov/iaui/894.02/related_projects/muc/proceedings/muc_7_toc.htm l).To evaluate the systems with a simple metric, two scores were defined, recall (3) and precision (4). The calculation of the scores is very similar for the different tasks except for the CO task. As an example we show the calculation of the scores for the TE task which are taken from the MUCs Scoring Software User's Manual. Two filled templates are compared, one filled manually which contains the *keys* and one filled by the software which contains *responses*.

Given the definitions:

- COR Correct - the two single fills are considered identical,
- INC Incorrect - the two single fills are not identical,
- PAR Partially Correct - the two single fills are not identical, but partial credit should still be given,
- MIS Missing - a key object has no response object aligned with it,
- SPU Spurious - a response object has no key object aligned with it,

- POS Possible - The number of fills in the key which contribute to the final score,
- ACT Actual - The number of fills in the response

the following values are calculated:

$$ACT = COR + INC + PAR + SPU . \tag{1}$$

$$POS = COR + INC + PAR + MIS . \tag{2}$$

$$REC = \frac{COR + 0.5 * PAR}{POS} . \tag{3}$$

$$PRE = \frac{COR + 0.5 * PAR}{ACT} . \tag{4}$$

van Rijsbergen's F-measure (5) is used to combine recall and precision measures into one measure. The formula for F is

$$F = \frac{(\beta^2 + 1) * PRE * REC}{(\beta^2 * PRE) + REC} . \tag{5}$$

The definitions for precision and recall found in the literature may differ slightly from those given above. Therefore it is recommended to be careful when applying these scores for comparing IE systems.

The Problem when Applying IE to the Biological Domain. The traditional IE tasks as specified in the MUCs are concerned with newspaper articles. Compared to these articles the structure of a sentence in the biological domain tends to be more complicated. Also the NE task is quite more challenging because of the confusing nomenclature of genetics. One gene often has more than one name or consists of a compound noun phrase. Additionally these noun phrases do not follow strict orthographical rules. For instance 'NFKB2' or 'nuclear factor of kappa light polypeptide gene enhancer in B-cells 2 (p49/p100)'or 'LYT-10' are synonyms for the same gene. And 'NF-kappa-b', 'nf-kappa-b' or 'NF Kappa B' presumably mean one and the same thing. Moreover, researchers studying different organisms have created quite different naming traditions. The Drosophila geneticists use such interesting names like "hedgehog" or "lost in space", while other communities name the genes after the molecular function of the protein they encode. "Biologists would rather share their toothbrush than share a genes name," said Michael Ashburner, head of the European Bioinformatics Institute in an interesting article in *Nature* about this subject [24]. All these problems call for sophisticated methods for name identification [25], [26], [27].

The task of identifying relations between genes is even more complicated because of the various linguistic forms one can express the relationship. The verbal phrases which represent the relationship may be nominalized or in passive form. Often several facts and relationships are concatenated or embedded in one sentence. Consider the following sentence:

These TD IkappaB mutants almost completely inhibited the induction of monocyte chemoattractant protein-1, interleukin-8, intercellular adhesion molecule-1, vascular cell adhesion molecule-1, and E-selectin expression by TNF-alpha, whereas interferon-gamma-mediated up-regulation of intercellular adhesion molecule-1 and HLA-DR was not affected [28].

The following biological reactions are expressed:
- Interferon-gamma mediates the up-regulation of intercellular adhesion melcule-1
- Interferon-gamma mediates the up-regulation of HLA-DR
- TD IkappaB mutants do NOT affect 1. and 2.
- TD IkappaB mutants inhibit the induction of monocyte chemoattractant protein-1 etc.

From this example it can be seen that complex semantical and syntactical analysis is needed to extract the relationships described by authors in the biomedical documents. Proposals in the literature how to handle this task range from simplifying assumptions to the use of full parsing.

The earlier works in this field concentrated on the task of extracting substance names and other terms to build dictionaries or ontologies. In recent research projects the focus shifted to extract information about interactions and relations between substances. For instance, [29] look for co-occurring gene names and assign those genes a relation if they co-occur with statistically significant frequency, leaving out the details of the relation. Much of the work reported so far focuses on extracting protein-protein interactions. [30] describe a system that extracts protein-protein interactions from MEDLINE abstracts. After locating the protein names, the system tries to find out the "actor" (subject) and the "patient" (object) of the proteins and thus also extracts the direction of the interaction. A very pragmatic approach is given by [31] with creation of a gene-to-gene co-citation network for 13712 human genes by automated analysis of titles and abstracts in over 10 million Medline records. [32] report on the adaptation of the general purpose IE system LaSIE to the biological domain. The resulting systems PASTA and EmPathIE extract information about protein structure and enzyme and metabolic pathway information respectively. [33] extract relations associated with the verbs *activate, bind, interact, regulate, encode, signal,* and *function*. The system from [34] only extracts protein interactions associated with the verb phrases *interact with, associate with,* and *bind to*. Another interesting approach is that of [35]. They report on the system GeneScene in which they use preposition-based templates combined with a word classification using WordNet 1.6. The average precision is 70 %. However, the method has some potential for improvement and moreover it is not restricted to proteins or genes as the agents and the verb phrases describing the interaction need not be pre-specified. [36] report on preliminary results on using a full parser for the extraction of events from the biomedical literature. An event can be viewed as activity or occurrence of interest e.g. a biological reaction. This task is quite more complex than the extraction of interactions because it identifies the dependencies or sequences of events.

The IE module in our software system is similar to the systems described above. But there is a main difference: in almost all of the projects mentioned above the extracted information is presented to the user in form of a structured representation. Our application goes a step further in that the extracted information is used to automatically construct a genetic network and thus contributes to the process of transformation of information into knowledge. There is no direct interaction with the user in which the result is controlled visually by the user. Information extraction systems often sacrifice precision for recall, or vice versa. If a system is tuned to have a good recall, it often extracts more than it should (bad precision). In our case, where the system should give an interpretation of the data this would possibly lead to a wrong hypothesis and may form the basis for further experiments. To avoid this problem our system should rather have a high precision than a high recall. It is more tolerable to miss a relation than to indicate a wrong relationship.

The last paragraph outlines the design of our IE module. The input to the IE module is a list of gene identifiers, i.e. genes classified by the neural network as a typical gene pattern. For each gene identifier a list of gene names and synonyms is generated using a precompiled dictionary. This set of synonyms is used as a basis for the search in the PubMed abstracts. Together with the synonyms a set of terms describing the causal relationship of genes is used to further specify the query. These terms are listed manually after analysing a set of relevant PubMed abstracts. For example the terms 'co-expressed' or 'co-regulated' are often used to describe the causal relationship we are looking for. The result of the query is a set of abstracts which is downloaded for further processing. The next step in the text analysis is to find and extract the information needed. To fulfil these tasks we have to go through several phases which contain more or less the tasks described above. The first phase can be described as a text-pre-processing phase. In this phase a tagger is used to put annotations to each word or symbol. These annotations are used in the subsequent steps to identify the predefined entities like gene or protein names. Once these entities are recognized, a set of rules is used to identify the relationship between the entities. In the last phase the extracted information is filled into pre-specified templates which are than transformed into database records. These database records are than used for the generation of genetic networks.

5 Visualization of Genetic Networks

Resulting genetic networks – consisting of a set of genes and causal relations between them - are presented in a static 3D structure by a visualization tool, which is developed in Inprise Delphi integrating the technology of OpenGL. Genes are presented as globes with expression labels or identifiers of relevant internet databases (members of tripartite: GenBank, EMBL and DDBJ or GeNet) to be chosen optionally. Genes will be linked by arrows if they are related. In future we will develop interactive components for users to choose a set of related genes and zoom into the genetic network. First results of utilizing several components of our software system separately are available. Networks of Drosophila and Sea Urchin we obtained from internet database GeNet information. Gene relation information for Drosophila and Sea Urchin are mined from

GeNet by our parser engine tool automatically: a special database adapter connects to GeNet and imports relevant html-pages with gene relation information for local storage, a local installed parser mines information about genes and gene-related regulatory connections from Drosophila and Sea Urchin. After parsing html-pages all data (genes and relations between them) can be presented by visualization tool as genetic network. The Drosophila network we obtained from GeNet database was compared with and is according to regulatory connection information of Drosophila genes online visible in GeNet. For Sea Urchin we couldn't get comparable maps from GeNet so far. The network of NFκB interactions (Fig. 4) is a composition of scientific publications [37], [38], [39].

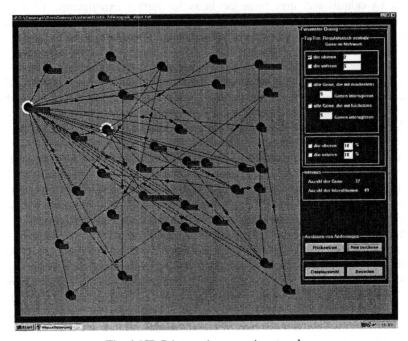

Fig. 4. NFκB interactions genetic network

Our visualization tool presents genetic networks in a static way. Labels give short information required to identify genes. The hint function of Delphi is used to describe gene identification in detail by text description, different identifiers and information source. To specify the relations between genes represented by lines we integrated several relation modes presented to the user by line modifications as arrows or colours. In this way an intuitive user interface is presented. Arrows show mode of causality: agent and target gene. The arrow colour gives more information: red stands for activation, blue for repression and grey stands for no specification.

Users have different options to single out very typical and pregnant genes in the considered disease association. One feature is the visual identification of regulatory central genes regarding the number of interactions with other genes by dying their direct background. Users can choose between absolute and relative approach optionally. They have the possibility to mark these regulatory central genes within a network by underlying them light (white markers). Otherwise it is possible to mark very inactive genes by underlying them dark (grey markers) in the same presentation. An interactive mode for graphical representing of genetic networks is advised in future to give users more efficient implements for understanding regulatory network. Given that to grasp the dynamic behaviour of cells under disease condition it is evident to understand the principles of regulatory genes networks organisation. And wouldn't be "learning by doing" with intuitive visualization the simplest way to succeed in understanding complex behaviour of cells?

6 Future Work – Integrating Methods of Case-Based-Reasoning (CBR)

In addition to neural network component ART1 we apply AI-methods of case-based-reasoning in our software system. As the technique of case-based-reasoning has been practised successfully in several domains like diagnostics, prediction, control and planning [40], [41] we want to utilize this technique for incremental modelling genetic networks. Each genetic network is considered as a case within the human genome. Similar cases represent similar genetic networks. Each stored identified case in the case base facilitates the retrieval of furthermore cases, i.e. genetic networks. The single cases have to be induced qualified for retrieving similar cases very fast and for integrating new cases into the case base, respectively. Inconsistence and incompleteness are characteristic features of genetic networks in consequence of incremental steady increase of knowledge about the human proteome. As a result the revise-phase is particularly important within the retrieval-reuse-revise-retain-loop of case-based-reasoning systems to control and revise the case base permanently. For this task a set of practicable techniques of our previous work [42] and according to the international level of research are available (e.g. contrast model by Tversky) [43], [44]. We will obtain a similarity tree of prototypes of genetic networks of different diseases. These prototypes will be represented by nodes of the similarity tree.
A similarity tree of experimental expression data is available from our previous work. The experimental data come from labs from Universities of Rostock, Bochum and Greifswald and from research institutes like DKFZ Heidelberg and Stanford. Nodes are representing autoimmune diseases like chronic pancreatitis, multiple sclerosis, rheumatic arthritis and further ones, but the focus is on actual research themes like autoimmune diseases. First genetic networks as nodes of similarity tree (*Drosophila*, Sea Urchin, intestinal inflammation or NFκB interactions as immune response in MS and RA) are generated with single software components developed at our institute, further ones like a genetic network of CP will follow soon. Available networks are nodes of similarity tree which have only one leaf up to now. In other words the node is in the same state as the leaf. These networks are to be considered as a start up and may demonstrate a prototype version of a software system for genomic data analysis.

7 Conclusions

Large-scale gene expression analysis is opening new perspectives in therapeutic research by providing objective global views of biological behaviour inside cells.

There are a few important points that should be considered when interpreting micro array gene expression data. We outlined some problems of data processing and statistical data analysis in the genomic data field and introduced a complex bioinformatic approach for processing genomic data and data mining to generate genetic networks as a complex answer to the complex genomic task.

Our straightforward future work will be focused on two principle tasks: first on practicing and linking AI-methods like neural ART-net and case-based learning methods and implementing them for categorizing diseases as well as second on successive increment of our case base for adapting existing networks and generating new ones. We have to practice a neural network and case-based learning methods with expression data mentioned in paragraphs 4 and 6 to realize our idea of generating nodes from more than one leaf in future. Results from preliminary investigations conducted with comparable data and neural ART-net tune us optimistically, that AI-methods are suitable to analyse array data for discovering disease typical gene patterns and in the accomplishment potentially target genes. In this context we will have to deal with questions like how to measure the similarity of genetic networks. We have to advance a sophisticated IE tool to mine gene relation information from public databases. Our system as a complex working software architecture will facilitate deciding diagnosis and therapy on the base of genomic knowledge and moreover discovering targets for drugs. Conventional methods of clustering excepting biological background knowledge don't suffice for that purpose.

References

1. Alter, O., Brown, P.O., Botstein, D.:Singular value decomposition for genome-wide expression data processing and modeling. PNAS **97**, Vol. 18 (2000) 10101-10106
2. Bassett, D.E.J.R., Eisen, M.B., Boguski, M.S.: Gene expression informatics – it's all in your mine. Nature Genetics Supplement **21** (1999) 51-55
3. Berry, M.J.A., Linoff, G.: Mining techniques for marketing, sales und customer support. John Wiley & Sons, New York (1997)
4. Eisen, M.B., Spellmann, P.T., Brown, P.O., Botstein, D.: Cluster analysis and display of genome-wide expression patterns. PNAS **95, Vol.** 25 (1998) 14863-14868
5. Duggan, D.J., Bittner, M., Chen, Y., Meltzer, P., Trent, J.M.: Expression profiling using cDNA microarrays. Nature **21** (1999) 10-14
6. Perner, P.: Classification of Hep-2 Cells using Fluorescent Image Analysis and Data Mining. In: Crespo, J., Maojo, V.,Martin, F. (eds.): Medical Data Analysis. (2001) 219-224
7. Chen, Y., Dougherty, E.R., Bittner, M.L.: Ratio-based decisions and the quantitative analysis of cDNA microarray images. J Biomed. Optics **2** (1997) 364-374
8. Oliver, S.: Guilt-by-association goes global. Nature **403** (2000) 601-603
9. Brazma, A., Hingamp, P., Quackenbush, J., Sherlock, G., Spellman, P., Stoeckert, C., Aach, J., Ansorge, W., Ball, C.A., Causton, H.C., Gaasterland, T., Glenisson, P., Holstege, F.C., Kim, I.F., Markowitz, V., Matese, J.C., Parkinson, H., Robinson, A., Sarkans, U., Schulze-Kremer, S., Stewart, J., Taylor, R., Vilo, J., Vingron, M.: Minimum information about microarray experiment (MIAME) towards standards for microarray data. Nature Genetics **29** Vol. 4 (2001) 365-371
10. Schena, M., Shalon, D., Davis, R.W., Brown, P.O.: Quantitative monitoring of gene expression patterns with a complementary DNA microarray. Science **270** (1995) 467-470

11. Velculescu, V.E., Zhang, L., Vogelstein, B., Kinzler, K.W.: Serial analysis of gene expression. Science **70** Vol. 5235 (1995) 484-487
12. Lockhart, D.J., Dong, H., Byrne, M.C., Follettie, M.T., Gallo, M.V., Chee, M.S., Mittmann, M., Wang, C., Kobayashi, M., Horton, H., Brown, E.L.: Expression monitoring by hybridization to high-density oligonucleotide arrays. Nat. Biotechnol. **14** (1996) 1675-1680
13. Ibrahim, S.M., Mix, E., Bottcher, T., Koczan, D., Gold, R., Rolfs, A., Thiesen, H.J.: Gene expression profiling of the nervous system in murine experimental autoimmune encephalomyelitis. Brain **124** (2001) 1927-1938
14. Everitt, B.S.: The Cambridge Dictionary of Statistics in the Medical Sciences. Cambridge University Press. (1995)
15. Khan, J., Simon, R., Bittner, M., Chen, Y., Leighton, S.B., Pohida, T., Smith, P.D., Jiang, Y., Gooden, G.C., Trent, J.M., Meltzer, P.S.: Gene expression profiling of alveolar rhabdomyosarcoma with cDNA microarrays. Cancer Res. **58** (1998) 5009-5013
16. Debouk, C. and Goodfellow, P.: DNA microarrays in drug discovery and development. Nature Genet. **21** (1999) 48-50
17. Glass, Ä.: A bioinformatic approach for generating genetic networks. Biosystems and Medical Technology **2** (2000) 52
18. Smaglik, P.: For my next trick. Nature **407** (2000) 828-829
19. Somogyi, R.: Making sense of gene-expression data. Pharmainformatics (1999) 17-24
20. Carpenter, G. A., Grossberg, S.: A massively parallel architecture for a self organizing neural pattern recognition machine. Computer Vision, Graphics, and Image processing **37** (1987) 54-115
21. Michel, E., Zernikow, B., Wichert, S.A.: Use of an artificial neural network (ANN) for classifying care needed, using incomplete input data. Med. Inform. **25** Vol. 2 (2000) 147-158
22. Kneller, D.G., Cohen, F.E., Langridge, R.: Improvements in protein secundary structure prediction by an enhanced neural network. J Mol Biol **214** (1990) 171-182
23. Wessel, M.D., Jurs, P.C., Tolan, J.W., Muskal, S.M.: Prediction of human intestinal absorption of drug compounds from molecular structure. J. Chem. Inf. Comput. Sci **38** Vol.4 (1998) 726-735
24. Pearson, H.: Biology`s name game. Nature **411** (2001) 631-632
25. Fukuda, K., Tsunoda, T., Tamura, A., Takagi, T.: Towards information extraction: Identifying protein names from biological papers. In Proc. 3rd Paci. Symposium of Biocomputing (1998) 707–718
26. Proux, D., Rechenmann, F., Julliard, L., Pillet, V., Jacq, B.: Detecting gene symbols and names in biological texts: A first step toward pertinent information extraction. In: Genome Informatics, Universal Academy Press (1998) 72–80
27. Krauthammer, M., Rzhetsky, A., Morozov, P., Friedman, C.: Using BLAST for identifying gene and protein names in journal articles. Gene **259** (2000) 245-252
28. Denk, A. J.: Activation of NF-kappa B via the Ikappa B kinase complex is both essential and sufficient for proinflammatory gene expression in primary endothelial cells. Biol Chem **30** Vol. 276 (2001) 28451-28458
29. Stapley, B., Benoit, G.: Biobibliometrics: information retrieval and visualization from co-occurrences of gene names in medline abstracts. Pacific Symposium on Biocomputing **5** (2000) 529-540
30. Wong, L.: PIES A Protein Interaction Extraction System. Pacific Symposium on Biocomputing **6** (2001)
31. Jenssen, T.K., Laegreid, A., Komorowski, J., Hovig, E.: A literature network of human genes for high-throughput analysis of gene expression. Nature Genetics **28** (2001) 21- 28
32. Humphreys, K., Demetriou, G., Gaizauskas, R.: Bioinformatics Applications of Information Extraction from Scientific Journal Articles. Journal of Information Science **26** Vol.2 (2000) 75-85

33. Sekimizu, T., Park, H., Tsujii, J.: Identifying the interaction between genes and gene products based on frequently seen verbs in MEDLINE abstracts. in Genome Informatics. Universal Academy Press, Inc. (1998)
34. Thomas, J., Milward, D., Ouzounis, C., Pulman, S., Carroll, M.: Automatic extraction of protein interactions from scientific abstracts. Pacific Symposium on Biocomputing **5** (2000) 538-549
35. Leroy, G., Chen, H.: Filling preposition-based templates to capture information from medical abstracts. Pacific Symposium on Biocomputing **7** (2002)
36. Yakushiji, A., Tateisi, Y., Miyao, Y., Tsujii, J.: Event Extraction from Biomedical Papers Using a Full Parser. Pacific Symposium on. Biocomputing, **6** (2001) 408-419
37. Miterski, B., Boehringer, S., Klein, W., Sindern, E., Haupts, M., Schimrigk, S., Epplen, J.T.: Inhibitors in the NFκB cascade comprise prime candidate genes predisposing to multiple sclerosis, especially in selected combinations, Genes and Immunity, (2002) in press.
38. Deng, L., Wang, C., Spencer, E., Yang, L., Braun, A., You, J., Slaughter, C., Pickart, C., Chen, Z.J.: Activation of the IkappaB kinase complex by TRAF6 requires a dimeric ubiquitin-conjugating enzyme complex and a unique polyubiquitin chain. Cell **103** Vol. 2 (2000) 351-361
39. Yang, J., Lin, Y., Guo, Z., Cheng, J., Huang, J., Deng, L., Liao, W., Cheng, Z., Liu, Zg., Su, B.: The essential role of MEKK3 in TNF-induced NF-kappaB activation. Nat Immunol **2** Vol. 7 (2001) 620-624
40. Heindl, B., Schmidt, R., Schmid, G., Haller, M., Pfaller, P., Gierl, L., Pollwein, B.: A Case-Based Consiliarius for Therapy Recommendation (ICONS): Computer-Based Advice for Calculated Antibiotic Therapy in Intensive Care Medicine. Computer Methods and Programs in Biomedicine **52** (1997) 117-127
41. Schmidt, R., Gierl, L.: Case-based reasoning for antibiotics therapy advice: an investigation of retrieval algorithms and prototypes. Artif Intel Med **23** 2001 171-186
42. Gierl, L., Bull, M., Schmidt, R.: CBR in Medicine. In: Bartsch-Spörl B, Wess S, Burkhard H-D, Lenz M (Hrsg.) Case-Based Reasoning Technology - from Foundation to Applications. Springer-Verlag, Berlin (1998) 273-297
43. Aamodt, A., Plaza, E.: Case-based reasoning: Foundational issues, methodological variations and system approaches. AICOM **7** Vol. 1 (1994) 39-59
44. Tversky, A.: Features of Similarity. Psychological Review **84** (1977) 327-352

Case-Based Reasoning for Prognosis of Threatening Influenza Waves

Rainer Schmidt and Lothar Gierl

Universität Rostock, Institut für Medizinische Informatik und Biometrie,
Rembrandtstr. 16 / 17, D-18055 Rostock, Germany
{rainer.schmidt/lothar.gierl}@medizin.uni-rostock.de

Abstract. The goal of the TeCoMed project is to compute early warnings against forthcoming waves or even epidemics of infectious diseases, especially of influenza, and to send them to interested practitioners, pharmacists etc. in the German federal state of Mecklenburg-Western Pomerania. Usually, each winter one influenza wave can be observed in Germany. In some years they are nearly unnoticeable, while in other years doctors and pharmacists even run out of vaccine. Because of the irregular cyclic behaviour it is insufficient to determine average values based on former years and to give warnings as soon as such values are noticeably overstepped. So, we have developed a method that combines Temporal Abstraction with Case-based Reasoning. The idea is to search for former, similar cases and to make use of them for the decision whether early warning is appropriate or not.

1   Introduction

The goal of our TeCoMed project is to compute early warnings against forthcoming waves or even epidemics of infectious diseases, especially of influenza, and to send them to interested practitioners, pharmacists etc. in the German federal state Mecklenburg-Western Pomerania. Available data are written confirmations of unfitness for work, which have to be sent by affected employees to their employers and to their health insurance companies. These confirmations contain the diagnoses made by their doctors. Since 1997 we receive these data from the main German health insurance company.

Many people believe influenza to be rather harmless. However, every year influenza virus attacks worldwide over 100 million people [1] and kills alone in the United States between 20.000 and 40.000 people [2]. The most lethal outbreak ever, the Spanish Flu in 1918, claimed 20-40 million lives worldwide, which is more than the second world war on both sides together [3].

In fact, influenza is the last of the classic plagues of the past which has yet to be brought under control [4]. Consequently, in the recent years some of the most developed countries have started to generate influenza surveillance systems (e.g. US: www.flustar.com, France [4], and Japan [5]).

Usually, each winter one influenza wave can be observed in Germany. However, the intensities of these waves vary very much. In some years they are nearly

P. Perner (Ed.): Advances in Data Mining 2002, LNAI 2394, pp. 99–107, 2002.

unnoticeable (e.g. in the winter of 1997/98), while in other years doctors and pharmacists even run out of vaccine (e.g. in the winter of 1995/96). Furthermore, figure 1 shows that influenza waves occurred in February and March. However, we know that this is probably accidental and in Germany a wave may already start much earlier (the last influenza epidemic started in December 1995).

Influenza waves are difficult to predict, because they are cyclic, but not regular [6]. Because of the irregular cyclic behaviour, it is insufficient to determine average values based on former years and to give warnings as soon as such values are noticeably overstepped. So, we have developed a method that combines Temporal Abstraction [7] with Case-based Reasoning [8, 9]. The idea is to search for former, similar courses and to make use of them for the decision whether early warning is appropriate.

Viboud et al. [10] apply the method of analogues [11], which originally was developed for weather forecasting. It also takes former, similar courses into account. However, the continuations of the most similar former courses are used to predict future values, e.g. the influenza incidences of next week. Instead, we intend to discover threatening influenza waves in advance and to provide early warnings against them.

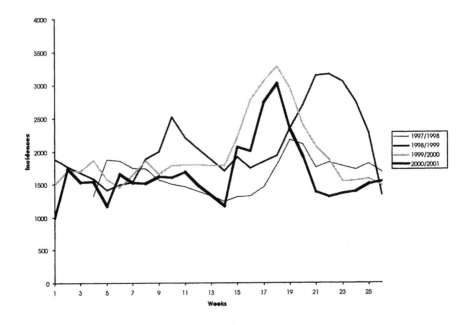

Fig. 1. Influenza courses for Mecklenburg-Western Pomerania from October till March. The 1st week corresponds to the 40th week of the calendar and 14th week to the 1st week of the next year.

2   Methods

Within the ICONS project we have already developed an early warning system, namely for the kidney function, which we have presented at last years MLDM conference [12] (for complete details see [13]). Our method concerning the kidney function combines Temporal Abstraction [7] with Case-based Reasoning [8, 9]. For predicting influenza waves, we apply the same ideas and methods again.

2.1   Case-Based Reasoning

Case-based Reasoning means to use previous experience represented as cases to understand and solve new problems. A case-based reasoner remembers former cases similar to the current problem and attempts to modify solutions of former cases to fit for the current problem. Figure 2. shows the Case-based Reasoning cycle developed by Aamodt and Plaza [14], which consists of four steps: retrieving former similar cases, adapting their solutions to the current problem, revising a proposed solution, and retaining new learned cases.

However, there are two main subtasks in Case-based Reasoning [14, 15]: The retrieval, the search for similar cases, and the adaptation, the modification of solutions of retrieved cases.

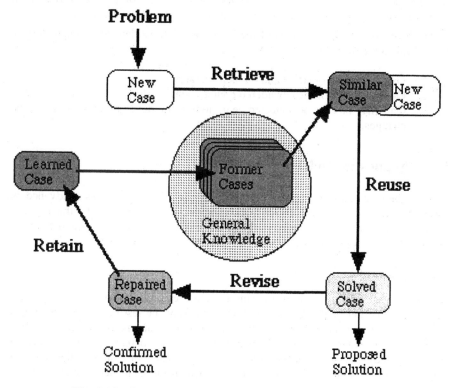

Fig. 2. The Case-based Reasoning cycle developed by Aamodt

Since differences between two cases are sometimes very complex, especially in medical domains, many case-based systems are so called retrieval-only systems. They just perform the retrieval task, visualise current and similar cases, and sometimes additionally point out the important differences between them [16]. Our early warning system for the kidney function [12, 13] just performs retrieval too.

2.2   Temporal Abstraction

Temporal Abstraction has become a hot topic in Medical Informatics in the recent years. For example, in the diabetes domain measured parameters can be abstracted into states (e.g. low, normal, high) and afterwards aggregated into intervals called episodes to generate a so-called modal day [17]. The main principles of Temporal Abstraction have been outlined by Shahar [7]. The idea is to describe a temporal sequence of values, actions or interactions in a more abstract form, which provides a tendency about the status of a patient. For example, for monitoring the kidney function it is fine to provide a daily report of multiple kidney function parameters. However, information about the development of the kidney function on time and, if appropriate, an early warning against a forthcoming kidney failure means a huge improvement [13].

To describe tendencies, an often-realised idea is to use different trend descriptions for different periods of time, e.g. short-term or long-term trend descriptions etc. [e.g. 16]. The lengths of each trend description can be fixed or they may depend on concrete values (e.g. successive equivalent states may be concatenated).

However, concrete definitions of the trend descriptions depend on characteristics of the application domain:

(1)   On the number of states and on their hierarchy,
(2)   On the lengths of the considered courses, and
(3)   On what has to be detected, e.g. long-term developments or short-term changes.

3   Prognostic Model for TeCoMed

Since we believe that warnings can be appropriate in about four weeks in advance, we consider courses that consist of four weekly incidences. However, so far this is just an assumption that might be changed in the future. Figure 3. shows the prognostic model for TeCoMed. It consists of four steps (the grey boxes on the right side).

3.1   Temporal Abstraction

We have defined three trends concerning the changes on time from last week to this week, from last but one week to this week, and from the last but two weeks to this week. The assessments for these three trends are "enormous decrease", "sharp decrease", "decrease", "steady", "increase", "sharp increase", and "enormous increase". They are based on the percentage of change. For example, the third, the long-term trend is assessed as "enormous increase" if the incidences are at least 50%

higher than those three weeks ago. If they are only at least 30% higher, it is assessed as "sharp increase", and if they are only at least 5% higher, it just an "increase".

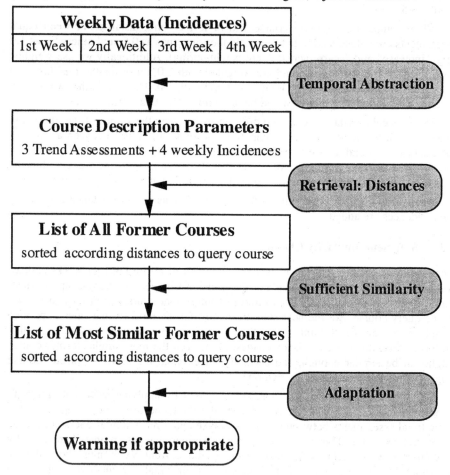

Fig. 3. The prognostic model for TeCoMed

Together with the four weekly data these assessments are used to determine similarities between a query course and all courses stored in the case base. Our intention for using these two sorts of parameters is to ensure that a query course and an appropriate similar course are on the same level (similar weekly data) and that they have similar changes on time (similar assessments).

3.2   Searching for Similar Courses

So far, we compute distances between a query course and all courses stored in the case base sequentially. In the future we hope to develop a more efficient retrieval algorithm. The considered attributes are the three nominal valued trend assessments and the four weekly incidences. The similarity measure is only based on our considerations, because no knowledge about it is available and learning by comparison with desired results is already necessary for a later step (explained in section 3.5.).

When comparing a current course with a former one, distances between equal assessments are valued as 0.0, between neighbouring ones as 0.5, and otherwise as 1.0 (e.g. "increase" and "sharp increase" are neighbouring). Additionally we use weights; the values for the short-term trend are weighted with 2.0, those for the medium-term trend with 1.5, and those for the long-term trend with 1.0. The idea is that we believe that more recent developments should be more important than earlier ones.

For the weekly data, we compute differences between the values of the query and those of each former course. We compute an absolute difference between a value of the query course and a value of a former course. Afterwards we divide the result by the value of the query course and weight it with the number of the week within the four weeks course (e.g. the first week gets the weight 1.0, the current week gets 4.0).

Finally, the distance concerning the trend assessments and the distance concerning the incidences are added.

3.3   Sufficient Similarity Check

The result of computing distances is a very long list of all former four weeks courses sorted according to their distances. For the decision whether a warning is appropriate, this list is not really helpful, because most of the former courses are rather dissimilar to the query course. So, the next step means to find the most similar ones. One idea might be to use a fixed number, e.g. the first two or three courses in the sorted list. Unfortunately, this has two disadvantages. First, even the most similar former course might not be similar enough, and secondly, vice versa, the fourth, fifth etc. course might be nearly as similar as the first one.

So, we decided to filter the most similar cases by applying sufficient similarity conditions. So far, we use just two thresholds. First, the difference concerning the three trend assessments between the query course and a most similar course has to be below a threshold X. This condition guarantees similar changes on time. And secondly the difference concerning the incidences of the current week must be below a threshold Y. This second condition guarantees an equal current level. Of course further conditions concerning the incidences of the three weeks ago might also be used.

3.4   Adaptation

So, now we have got a usually very small list that contains only the most similar former courses. However, the question arises how these courses can help to decide whether early warning is appropriate. In Case-based Reasoning, the retrieval usually provides just the most similar case whose solution has to be adapted to fit for the query course. As in Compositional Adaptation [19] we take the solutions of a couple of similar cases into account.

The question is: what are the solutions of courses of incidences? The obvious idea is to treat the course continuation of a four weeks course as its solution. However, in contrast to Viboud et al. [10] we do not intend to predict future incidences, but to provide interested people (practitioners, pharmacists etc.) with warnings against approaching influenza waves. So, we have marked those time points of the former courses where we, in retrospect, believed a warning would have been appropriate; e.g. in the 17th week of the 2000/2001 season (see fig.1). This means that a solution of a four weeks course is a binary mark, either a warning was appropriate or not.

For the decision to warn, we split the list of the most similar courses in two lists. One list contains courses where a warning was appropriate; the second list gets the other ones. For both of these new lists we compute their sums of the reciprocal distances of their courses to get sums of similarities. Subsequently, the decision about the appropriateness of a warning depends on the question which of these two sums is bigger.

3.5   Learning

In section 3.3. we have introduced two threshold parameters X and Y. However, we have not explained how we are getting good settings for them. In fact there is no chance to know them. Since they are very important for the solution, namely the decision whether to warn, we attempt to learn them. For each of our complete influenza courses (from October to March), we have made the same experiment; we used it as query course and we have tried to compute the desired warnings with the remaining courses as case base. Therefor we have varied the values for the threshold parameters X and Y. So far, we have not learnt single optimal values but intervals for the threshold parameters. With combinations of values within these intervals all desired warnings can be computed.

4   First Results

So far, we have developed a program that computes early warnings of approaching influenza waves for the German federal state Mecklenburg-Western Pomerania. As we receive data since 1997, our case base just contains four influenza periods. For each of them, our program is able to compute the desired warnings by using the other three periods as case base. However, the last influenza epidemic in Western Europe, where doctors even ran out of vaccine, occurred in winter 1995-96 [20]. Unfortunately, we do not have data for this period. Nevertheless, we hope to be able to predict such epidemics with the help of our data of the recent influenza waves.

At present the computed warnings and follow-up warnings are only displayed on a machine. In the near future we intend to send them by email to interested people.

Furthermore, so far we have focussed on the temporal aspect of influenza waves for the whole federal state. Very recently, we have started to apply our program to smaller units, namely to 6 cities or towns and to 12 districts in Mecklenburg-Western Pomerania. Since we only receive data of written unfitness for work from the main health insurance company, incidences for some of these units are rather small (even the peaks are sometimes below 100 per week). For such units our program has difficulties to determine whether an increase is already the beginning of an influenza wave or if it occurred just accidentally. The general problem is that the smaller the incidences are, the higher is the influence of coincidence.

In the future, we additionally intend to study the geographical spread of influenza in Mecklenburg-Western Pomerania, although it seems to be difficult to determine the way epidemics spread in space [4, 20]. Furthermore, we plan to extend our research to further diseases, e.g. to bronchitis and to salmonellae.

References

1. Nichol, K.L. et al.: The effectiveness of Vaccination against Influenza in Adults. New England Journal of Medicine **333** (1995) 889-893
2. Hwang, M.Y.: Do you have the flu? JAMA **281** (1999) 962
3. Dowdle, W.R.: Informed Consent Nelson-Hall, Inc. Chicago, III
4. Prou, M., Long, A., Wilson, M., Jacquez, G., Wackernagel, H., Carrat, F.: Exploratory Temporal-Spatial Analysis of Influenza Epidemics in France. In: Flahault, A., Viboud, C., Toubiana, L., Valleron, A.-J.: Abstracts of the 3rd International Workshop on Geography and Medicine, Paris, October 17-19 (2001) 17
5. Shindo, N. et al.: Distribution of the Influenza Warning Map by Internet. In: Flahault, A., Viboud, C., Toubiana, L., Valleron, A.-J.: Abstracts of the 3rd International Workshop on Geography and Medicine, Paris, October 17-19 (2001) 16
6. Farrington, C.P., Beale, A.D.: The Detection of Outbreaks of Infectious Disease. In Gierl, L., Cliff, A.D., Valleron, A.-J., Farrington, P., Bull, M. (eds.): GEOMED '97, International Workshop on Geomedical Systems, Teubner-Verlag, Stuttgart Leipzig (1997) 97-117
7. Shahar, Y.: A Framework for Knowledge-Based Temporal Abstraction. Artificial Intelligence **90** (1997) 79-133
8. Lenz, M., Bartsch-Spörl, B., Burkhard, H.-D., Wess, S. (eds.): Case-Based Reasoning Technology, Lecture Notes in Artificial Intelligence, Vol. 1400. Springer-Verlag, Berlin Heidelberg New York (1998)
9. Perner, P.: Are Case-Based Reasoning and Dissimilarity-Based Classification Two Sides of the Same Coin? In: Perner, P. (eds.): Machine Learning and Data Mining in Pattern Recognition, Lecture Notes in Artificial Intelligence, Vol. 2123. Springer-Verlag, Berlin Heidelberg New York (2001) 35-51
10. Viboud, C., Boelle, P.-Y., Carrat, F., Valleron, A.-J., Flahault, A.: Forecasting the spatio-temporal spread of influenza epidemics by the method of analogues. In: Abstracts of the 22nd Annual Conference of the International Society of Clinical Biostatistics, Stockholm, August 20-24 (2001) 71
11. Lorenz, E.N.: Atmospheric predictability as revealed by naturally occuring analogies. J Atmos Sci (1969) 26
12. Schmidt, R., Gierl, L.: Temporal Abstractions and Case-Based Reasoning for Medical Course Data: Two Prognostic Applications. In: Perner, P. (eds.): Machine Learning and Data Mining in Pattern Recognition, Lecture Notes in Artificial Intelligence, Vol. 2123. Springer-Verlag, Berlin Heidelberg New York (2001) 23-34
13. Schmidt, R., Pollwein, B., Gierl, L.: Medical multiparametric time course prognoses applied to kidney function assessments. Int J of Medical Informatics **53** (2-3) (1999) 253-264
14. Aamodt, A., Plaza, E.: Case-based reasoning: Foundation issues. Methodological variation- and system approaches. AI Comunications 7(1) (1994) 39-59
15. Kolodner, J.: Case-Based Reasoning. Morgan Kaufmann Publishers, San Mateo (1993)
16. Macura, R., Macura, K.: MacRad: Radiology image resources with a case-based retrieval system. In: Aamodt, A., Veloso, M. (eds.): Case-Based Reasoning Research and Development, Proceedings of ICCBR-95, Lecture Notes in Artificial Intelligence, Vol. 1010. Springer-Verlag, Berlin Heidelberg New York (1995) 43-54

17. Larizza, C., Bellazzi, R., Riva, A.: Temporal abstraction for diabetic patients management. In: Keravnou, E., Garbay, C., Baud, R., Wyatt, J. (eds.): Proceedings of the 6th Conference on Artificial Intelligence in Medicine (AIME-97), Lecture Notes in Artificial Intelligence, Vol. 1211. Springer-Verlag, Berlin Heidelberg New York (1997) 319-330

18. Miksch, S., Horn, W., Popow, C., Paky, F.: Therapy planning using qualitative trend descriptions. In: Barahona, P., Stefanelli, M., Wyatt, J. (eds.): Proceedings of the 5th Conference on Artificial Intelligence in Medicine (AIME-95), Lecture Notes in Artificial Intelligence, Vol. 934. Springer-Verlag, Berlin Heidelberg New York (1995) 197-208

19. Wilke, W., Smyth, B., Cunningham, P.: Using Configuration Techniques for Adaptation. In: [8] 139-168

20. Carrat, F., Flahault, A., Boussard, E., Farron, N., Dangoumau, L., Valleron, A.-J.: Surveillance of influenza-like illness in France: The example of the 1995-96 epidemic. Journal of Epidemiology Community Health 52 (Suppl1) (1998) 32-38

Author Index

Druck und Bindung: Strauss GmbH, Mörlenbach

Lecture Notes in Artificial Intelligence (LNAI)

Lecture Notes in Computer Science